#ONECHOICE

#ONECHOICE

How Ten Seconds Can Change Your Life

NICK AND JACK SAVAGE

As told by their mom Becky

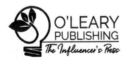

O'LEARY
PUBLISHING
The Influencer's Press

NAPLES, FL

ISBN (paperback): 978-1-952491-30-6
ISBN (hardcover):978-1-952491-39-9
ISBN (ebook): 978-1-952491-31-3
Library of Congress Control Number: 2021913147

Editing by Heather Davis Desrocher
Proofreading by Boris Boland
Book Design by Jessica Angerstein

Printed in the United States of America

To Mike, Nick, Jack, Justin and Matthew...

I love you more, always.

Goodbyes hurt the most
when the story was not finished.

–UNKNOWN

This Book is Presented By:

THE 525 FOUNDATION

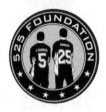

PREVENTING LOSS THROUGH
EDUCATION AND AWARENESS

The 525 Foundation exists to educate teens and families, and to raise awareness about the dangers of alcohol and prescription drug misuse and abuse.

We cannot do it without your help!

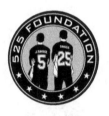

⬇ DOWNLOAD NOW

- #ONECHOICE Teacher-Student Study Guide

- Sample Conversation Starters

- Prevention resources and much more at:

www.525foundation.org

CONTENTS

Becky
(aka Mom)

The death of a child is so painful,
both emotionally and spiritually, that
I truly wondered if my own heart and
spirit would ever heal. I soon learned that
I could help myself best by helping others.

—BARBARA BUSH

Our lives were forever changed in the early morning hours of Sunday, June 14, 2015, when my two oldest sons – Nick and Jack – both died of an accidental overdose of oxycodone and alcohol. They were just 18 and 19 years old. Jack, a handsome, athletic, adventurous, young man, had just graduated from high school a week earlier, and was on his way to Ball State University to major in business. Nick, the oldest of my four boys, also handsome and adventurous, had a quick wit and a bit of shyness. He had just finished his freshman year of college at Indiana University in Bloomington, where he was majoring in chemistry and microbiology. They both had hearts of gold and had lived such full lives up to that point. They still had a lot more life to live. But all of their dreams – and ours – were gone in an instant.

I do not know why Nick and Jack made the choice to take someone else's prescription medication that fatal night in June. It was so unlike them. I am pretty sure that was not the first time that they ever had a beer, but I am almost certain that was the first time they had ever tried pills. In fact, Nick had a hard time swallowing any kind of pill or medicine. So, it was rare for him to even ask for something as basic as Tylenol or Advil – even for a splitting headache. And when he did ask for something, it was for the liquid form.

Did he, or someone else, crush up the pill in order for him to swallow it?

Either way, that night both Nick and Jack had hydrocodone in their system. The toxicology reports concluded that they also had alcohol in their systems, and that those two combined caused a fatal reaction in both of my boys – an overdose. It was an accidental overdose.

Their choice to take opioids that night will always haunt me. *Why did they take the pills? What were they thinking? Why didn't one of them stop the other?* My boys were "thick as thieves," and usually always watched out for the other. So their decision that night still haunts me.

Nick and Jack had a special sibling relationship admired by many. They were also looked upon as leaders in many of the crowds they hung out with, and they were looked up to in their wide circle of friends. This kind of choice was not like them.

In fact, I was with them for the first of a string of graduation parties that evening on Saturday, June 13, 2015. We were at Ryan's party first – Ryan was their friend and hockey teammate. I remember sitting under the white party tent in Ryan's backyard with a few other parents, watching my boys play cornhole with their friends. I remember thinking just how proud I was of both of them – proud of the way they treated people, the way they looked people in the eye during conversation, the respectful way they shook hands, the way they expressed their gratitude for being invited to the party, and the way they reacted to the well-wishes tossed their way.

I thought how handsome they both were – Jack with his blueish-green eyes, brown hair and slightly crooked, boyish smile, and Nick with his blue eyes, blonde hair, his long, tan legs, and gentle facial features. That night, Jack was wearing the new blue-and-white-striped golf polo shirt and Sperry shoes I bought for him, along with his typical khaki shorts. Nick had on a new plaid shirt and similar Sperry shoes and khaki shorts. That was their typical dress-up attire. I find it strange that I can remember these details so clearly, down to the slightest detail (what a blessing), considering there are so many things I can't remember.

My boys could be the life of the party and they always tried to make sure everyone was included in their laughter and fun – especially that night. And boy, did we have fun together!

As much as they teased and picked on each other, my boys loved each other. And they were always looking out for one another. *So, what made them think it was OK to pop someone else's prescription medication that night?*

We had the usual "talks" with our boys during their teenage years about illicit drugs, drinking and driving, and sex. I have been a nurse my entire adult life, so those kinds of conversations were second nature to me. They would shake their heads and raise their hands to signal the end of the conversation – or just the end of their listening.

But it never crossed my mind to talk to them about the dangers of opioids and prescription pills – especially **someone else's pills**. Talking to them about misusing prescription medications was not on our radar. We had no idea that teens were doing that sort of thing. And for heaven's sake, it was my job as a nurse to educate people on those kinds of choices. But we cannot educate on, or bring awareness to, something we do not know about.

I know I cannot dwell there. I cannot stay in the **"whys"** and **"what-ifs"** for too long. I have to keep moving forward. I owe it to my husband, Mike, and our two younger sons, Justin and Matthew, to keep moving forward – we have to keep moving forward as a family. That is why we created the 525 Foundation after Nick and Jack's deaths, using their hockey jersey numbers, 5 and 25. **The mission of our foundation is to educate teens and families and raise awareness**

about the dangers of alcohol and prescription drug misuse and abuse. This is called primary prevention.

Nick and Jack brought so much love and goodness to the world when they were alive. This book is my way of carrying on their legacy of love and goodness – by telling their story and about what happened that night. It is my way of trying to prevent another tragedy like the one that forever changed our lives.

As you read, consider the choice that Nick and Jack made. How did two brothers end up making the *One Choice* that ended their lives? How can you choose differently?

This is their story – the story of Nick and Jack Savage – as told by me, their mom.

It is narrated in their own voices, and is inspired by their lives and their brotherly love.

A SPECIAL NOTE

The purpose of this book is to tell Nick and Jack's story. #OneChoice honors the "do good" legacies they left behind in this world. We hope that this story will help prevent future accidental overdoses on prescription pills. We are not experts in the field – we just have experience in the field, and we hope this book will make a difference in the lives of those who read it.

THE EARLY YEARS
2000-2007

Nick

Childhood is the one story that
stands by itself in every soul.

—UNKNOWN

By kindergarten and first grade, I had moved past
the Barney phase. (Yes, the big purple dinosaur.
Embarrassing, I know.) Jack was ready to move on
from the Teletubbies, and I dove head first into Legos
and books. I loved anything to do with Pokemon
cards (including the Battle Box), Magic Treehouse
stories, and dragons. I was quick with the answers

in class, but quietly waited for my teachers to call on me before I would speak up. By now, I am sure you can guess that Jack was quite the opposite. If Jack knew the answer to a question, as he often did, he would just blurt it out. When that kind of thing happened, students like me who were quietly waiting for the teacher to call on them would slowly lower their hands in disappointment and wait to see if they knew the answer to the next question.

My favorite food was tacos, but I considered it a special occasion when we went to Chuck E. Cheese for pizza with friends or for a classmate's birthday party.

Around the same time, we moved to Woodington Court in Granger, in a home on the edge of the cul-de-sac. There were a ton of kids around our age living in that neighborhood, and many of them were boys. When we moved to that house, we ditched the appliance-sized cardboard boxes that we used to spend hours playing in as toddlers. Instead, we spent our days riding bikes, shooting hoops, playing games such as kickball or kick-the-can, and looking for frogs in the retention pond nearby. The parents all took turns providing snacks, since it would have been a waste of our playtime for each of us to stop what we were doing and run home to our houses to grab a snack every time we were hungry. We were affectionately known as the "Cul-de-sac Kids." And when we were not out front in the cul-de-sac, we were playing on the swing set or jumping on the trampoline in the backyard.

During the second week of school in second grade, Mom had another baby. On September 5, 2003, she brought home our baby brother and her fourth boy, Matthew Paul Savage. Like every other kid in our family, we called him a slew of nicknames, including Chunks. But Matty was the one that stuck as he got older – thank God. I was not that into babies, but I really loved that kid. Even to this day, Mom often says she sees a lot of me and Jack in Matty's personality. Maybe it was because we were old enough to help her, or read books to him before bedtime, but that kid seemed to be the best mix of the rest of us – Jack, Justin, and me.

Our elementary school was down the street and around the corner. And we hit the big time in fifth grade when we were allowed to ride our bikes to school with a helmet. Fifth grade was the school's rule. But of course, Jack broke that rule by riding his bike with me when I was in fifth grade and he was in fourth. All the teachers knew it, but all Jack had to do was flash his innocent crooked-smirk-smile, and no one had the heart to tell him he had to wait until the following year. I still remember him tossing his hair off to the side with a quick flick of his head, so he could strap his helmet on tight and still see past his bangs. We all had longer locks in those days. It was what Mom referred to as our "hockey hair."

I do not always remember the exact timeline of events from those early elementary school years. What I remember, instead, are the experiences and the fun times. I remember hanging out with my best pal, Nic Mensick. I remember doing the Learn-to-

Skate program at the Ice Box, the local ice rink in the neighboring town of South Bend. By the next year, I learned to play hockey. I was probably 6 or 7 years old at the time. My buddy Nic was playing with me, and Dad (Mike) was our coach. Jack played hockey too, but we were always on different teams because of the way our birthdays fell on the calendar.

I remember trying baseball for a few years, and my face still aches when I think about the time I got clocked with a ball during pregame warmups by the biggest kid on the team. It hurt like hell, but I did not want to show it. I stood up, shook my head to regain my composure, wiped the blood from my face with the backside of my sleeve, and kept tossing the ball back and forth. I was into basketball too, and spent hours shooting hoops in our cul-de-sac with some of the neighbor kids.

Later on in elementary school, I discovered history, math, science, and especially chemistry. I spent hours working on fun experiments and thumbing through the latest *Ripley's Believe It or Not* book or *Guinness*

Book of World Records from the school library. I once did a science fair project on germs, and got invited to display my project at the University of Notre Dame's local science fair.

I loved dogs and was obsessed with sharks. We always had a family dog that we adored – Duke, Scout, and Tucker. And at one point, I had a pet fish, which I proudly named Azul because he was blue and I was in the middle of learning my colors in Spanish at school. Azul is the Spanish word for blue.

Although it is unrelated to having pets but totally related to that stage of my life, I remember thinking, *When I grow up, I am going to be a policeman or race car driver.* I was timid, playful, curious and quietly adventurous as a kid. I am not sure that much has changed since then.

CHAPTER 2

Jack

Not to change anything,
but to feel a few things twice ...

—UNKNOWN

Nick already spilled the beans about the Teletubbies. I am not going to lie; I was slightly obsessed with *The Big Comfy Couch* and the song that went along with it. Thank God that phase did not last too long. And if anyone ever brings it up, I just blame it on Mom.

Speaking of Mom, Becky was always into big parties with crazy themes. We had some of the coolest birthday cakes, thanks to her obsession with trying to "make memories." There was the "magic" birthday party when I turned 5, complete with a real magician who put on a magic show in the basement. There was the baseball-cap cake for my 6th birthday. And the tall tower cake for my seventh birthday (that did not stay together long enough to hold my birthday candles, because it split in two when Mom pulled it from the refrigerator). Beck spent all afternoon the day before baking layers of cake to stack into a tower, but it was a complete failure. We laughed and laughed, although she didn't think it was funny. At least the cake tasted good!

Nick was born on Thanksgiving and was always a simple kind of guy, so his choice for birthday cakes matched his personality. It was pumpkin pie, plain and simple. For an extra-fancy treat, Mom would add a big scoop of Cool Whip to each slice. That was how

Nick preferred to celebrate his birthday – in a simple kind of way, for a simple kind of guy.

We both sang in the choir at school. I even had a solo part the year we did Elvis Presley's 1950s hit, "Jailhouse Rock." And there sat Beck, in the front row, cheering me on.

Nick, Justin and I wrestled nonstop with each other at home. Justin was just two years younger than I was, so he would wait until Nick and I were tangled up on the floor; then, he would jump on top of the pile. Nick loved to play Xbox with his friends. I was not as into video games as he was, but I paid attention to everything he did. I still remember the first time Nick hooked up the Xbox; we could hear my cousin's voice come over the speaker from his own bedroom, which was pretty cool because he lived all the way in Grand Rapids, a solid two hours from our house.

Mom would make a big breakfast on Sundays. And it was our job to clear the table and take care of the dishes after every family meal. I remember rushing through the cleanup so I could go back outside. I loved being outside with my friends. Mom said that when she would peek out the window or open the door to check on us, I was always laughing with my friends, or standing there grinning and watching my big brother. She said that nothing seemed to get me down, that I was always a happy kid with a can-do attitude. I loved a good challenge and was always up for adventure. "Yep, I'll go!" or "Yep, I'll do it!" were the phrases that most often came out of my mouth in those years. And I **loved** sports. Any sport. Give me a ball and a glove, or a basketball, or a lacrosse stick, or a hockey stick and puck, and I was good and quick. I just had a special knack for sports.

Nick and I rode the bus together to school every day until we were old enough to ride our bikes. I have fun memories of waiting at the bus stop with Nick and our neighborhood friends. We had the same bus driver all throughout elementary school. Her name was Jeanie, and she always greeted us with a smile. Nick and I shared a few teachers throughout elementary school, too. We especially loved Mrs. Young in fourth grade and Mrs. Haverstick in fifth grade. What I loved most about those two is that they were fun and engaging. Even though they knew that Nick and I were brothers, they never expected me to be like Nick. They gave me the freedom and permission to be my own Savage self.

Mrs. Young saved one of my assignments from the beginning of school that year, in September 2006, and gave it to my mom. We were learning how to write letters, and mine read:

> Dear Grampa Harry,
>
> You are specil to me because almost every time I came over with my brothers you would billed a bassdall bimand in your back yard so we could play bassdall. Thank you for dowing that. That was vary specil.
>
> I love you,
> Jack S.

Fourth grade with Mrs. Young was the year I had to put in some after-school hours with a few other kids to strengthen our reading and writing skills (obviously, as seen in the letter to "Grampa"). After the rest of our class was dismissed in groups of bus riders, bike-riders, and walkers, Mrs. Young gathered the remaining few on the floor by the chalkboard. We'd have a snack, then we would read together and talk about the lesson she was teaching that day. One late winter afternoon, I decided I could not concentrate until I did something with the bulky winter jacket laying on the floor next to me. So, I took off my shoes, stuck my legs through the armholes of the jacket and sat perfectly still, ready to learn, for the rest of our time together. Mrs. Young glanced at me with wide eyes, and when she saw I had settled in and was not going to be a jokester about it, she smiled and started the lesson.

I liked school well enough to earn good grades. But it was Nick who took his studies seriously during those elementary school days. Mom would take us to

Barnes & Noble bookstore on occasion and say, "Go ahead and pick out two books, boys. But just two!" Nick often convinced her to buy the three or four books he had under his arm, having spent 30 minutes combing the shelves. When the Scholastic book fair rolled through town, Mom would give us each $15 to spend. I spent at least half my cash on posters, games, and the 3-foot-long pencils they sold at the checkout; Nick spent all of his money on encyclopedias for kids, or "smart books," as I called them. Those were the kind of books that documented data and details for kids. I swear that he knew everything about sharks, and he would rattle off facts during Discovery's shark week while we watched programs after school.

At some point, I started calling Nick "Rule Book Rex" – I knew it annoyed him, but seriously, the kid knew everything, and he always tried to impress everyone by always following the rules. Geesh! But I loved him anyway.

The summer I turned 7, and Nick was still 8, Mom and Dad bought the lake house at Donnell Lake in southern Michigan, just a short 30-minute drive from home. Dad grew up going to that lake. In fact, some of his friends from elementary school still live on the lake today. Summers at the lake were some of my favorite memories as a kid. Dad would take us out fishing in the morning, and sometimes again at night, before we went to bed. Truth be told, he was probably giving Mom a break. Nick, Justin and I slept in the bunk room. It had two sets of bunk beds and was on a separate floor from Mom and Dad's room. That meant we could stay up talking, laughing and goofing around, long hours after they went to bed. When Matty was old enough to sleep in his own bed, he joined us in the bunk room too. Our days were filled with boating, fishing, wake-surfing, swimming – and eventually, dirt bike racing. And our nights were filled with campfires, s'mores, flashlight tag, card games and conversation.

The first summer we had the lakehouse, I played baseball. Mom and Dad made it work, driving back and forth between the lake and the baseball diamond near our home in Granger for practices and games. But by the time our second summer at the lake rolled around, I did not want to miss a single second of fun with my brothers, so I decided to give up baseball.

I remember going to Disney a few times during those early years. Mom and Dad had different kinds of vacation experiences when they were young, and they did their best to make special memories for us by taking us to fun places every once in a while. One time at Disney World in Florida, one of our cousins got lost because he wandered off to another area of the theme park without anyone noticing. It scared the hell out of Nick. Justin, Nick and I were trading Disney pins with the Disney characters and employees around the park. Justin and I kept running off, excited to trade our pins. But Nick always stayed within a safe radius and kept a close eye on Mom and Dad, even on the rare occasions when they were not keeping a close eye on us.

I was inquisitive, happy-go-lucky, daring, outgoing and adventurous as a kid. I am not sure much has changed.

COMING OF AGE
2008-2011

Nick

The deepest definition of youth
is life as yet untouched by tragedy.

— ALFRED NORTH WHITEHEAD

Our middle school years were a big deal. There was school and hockey and racing; dirt bikes and boats and duck hunting. We still spent most of our summers at the lake, and weekends there in the fall and spring, when the weather was warm. Mom still went all-out for our birthdays, and we spent a lot of time with our cousins and friends. Mom also went back to work full-time as a nurse educator. The trade-off was that spring break became our family thing. We often spent spring break somewhere on a beach in Sarasota, Florida, with family and friends.

Jack and I started getting more serious with hockey, and we both made our age group travel team in the IYHL (Indiana Youth Hockey League) with the Irish Rovers. I was not the best player and did not get a lot of playing time, but I loved being a part of the team. Jack was still on a different team due to our birthdays, which was a bummer.

When I started traveling for hockey, we spent most winter and early spring weekends in a nearby city: Chicago, Indianapolis, Detroit, Grand Rapids, and so on. Dad was always coaching one of our teams, which meant Mom was on weekend hockey duty for whichever one of us did not have Dad as a coach. Our little brothers were always in tow. On rare occasions, Jack's team and my team were in the same city or hosting tournaments back in South Bend.

CHAPTER 3

We played between the Ice Box and the newly-finished Compton Family Arena on the campus of Notre Dame. I still remember the game that Dad affectionately calls my "breakout game." I was on the Irish Rovers Peewee travel team, and we were playing down in Fort Wayne for the weekend. Dad helped coach that team, and it was always a comfort knowing that he was behind the bench. Our head coach put me at the center position for one of the shifts out on the ice during a mid-tournament game. I was nervous as heck because I usually played wing, but we were ahead on the scoreboard, so Coach decided to switch up a few things – including my position for a shift. Much to my surprise, and perhaps to the surprise of my teammates and our fans in the stands, I played really well. I was swift, strong and in a good position to move the puck around in front of the opposing team's goal. I was so proud of myself, and I am sure it showed. My smile was a mile wide behind that helmet and face shield.

One weekend, Jack happened to be traveling for hockey with Dad and me, while Mom went to pick out a white-yellow lab puppy. She Facetimed us when she got to the puppy place so we could help her pick out the dog. It was obvious that she wanted the quiet, small female in the litter; but we could already tell that we loved the biggest male, even through the phone screen. He was the most aggressive and outgoing of the bunch, and he made us laugh just watching him play around with his litter mates. It took Mom forever to decide, but she finally caved and came home with our favorite pick. We named him Tucker, and soon he was affectionately known as "Tuck." Tucker became a best friend to all of us – even my mom!

When we were not in school or on the ice, we were at the lake. Our lake house was one of our "happiest places on earth." We spent a lot of time up there, and we loved every minute of it. I was a cautious kid for the most part, but I was usually living vicarious adventures through the books I read – until Jack was old enough and persuasive enough to talk me into mischief. It was not bad mischief – I guess you would just call it pushing the envelope a bit.

It did not take much for him to convince me to ride my dirt bike without a helmet or swim without a life jacket when the grownups were not watching. But I learned quickly that Mom and Dad meant business when they said, "No life jacket, no boat ride." I told myself I would never again be left behind standing on the shore by myself, just because I refused to wear a life jacket. There were some rules my parents would not bend on, and I realized that a life jacket was one of those things. When we each turned 13, if we wanted to drive a boat, we had to take the boating safety class. Again, a rule that my parents would not bend on. So, we all took the course, and we all got to drive our family pontoon. I have to say it was well worth it – oh, the fun we had on that pontoon!

Late-night conversations in the bunk room at the lake house got louder and rowdier as we got older. Mom or Dad would pop in to ask us to quiet down and go to sleep. So we would pretend we were doing just that – going to sleep – for a solid minute or two, before we would go right back to talking, making loud noises, and giggling into the early hours of the morning. Our middle school friends – many of whom were part of our lake "family" – would occasionally spend a night or two in the bunk room with us. And at one point, my entire hockey team slept there, too. Like I said, the lake house was one of the happiest (and funnest) places in my world!

Jack was more of a daredevil in middle school than ever before. I am sure that my eyes were as big as saucers the night he lit a paper napkin on fire up at the lake, just to see how quickly it could burn. Well, it burned quickly, and without thinking, he tossed it into the trash can. I played the mature big brother role by checking to make sure the napkin burned out without catching anything else on fire, but it did! The trash was on fire; we ran the can outside and hosed it off. Whoa! *That was close*, I thought; I *don't think we will need to be doing that again!* Well, that was until the Fourth of July; the Fourth was like heaven for us kids. It was a free license to light things on fire and blow things up. But we always stayed safe (well, mostly), and knew we had Nurse Becky as a backup plan, just in case something went wrong.

Now working full-time during the week, Beck stayed home on weekends when Dad would take us up to one of the racetracks in southwest Michigan with our Grandpa Larry, Uncle Dave, and our cousin, Jameson. We'd pull a camper up there and stay at Grattan or GingerMan or RoadAmerica for a few days. Grandpa and Uncle Dave raced a yellow Lotus at some of the races.

And in between racetrack lineups, we would catch box turtles and frogs in a dirty pond nearby and play games with our cousins. At bedtime, we slept in the camper, or in a tent right outside the camper. On occasion, we even slept in the car. We'd roast hot dogs and marshmallows over the evening campfire – me with my Flamin' Hot Cheetos and Jack with his blue Gatorade and Sour Patch Kids. If we were at the races on a weekend close to Jack's birthday in late

May, Grandma would bake a cake and we'd have a party at our campsite.

I found a new love in middle school: **music.** I played the saxophone for one year in the middle school band. But that is not the kind of music I am referring to – I mean **real** music. At first, I liked bands with a heavy beat: AC/DC, Aerosmith and Led Zeppelin. But later in high school, my penchant for a heavy beat translated to rap music, and eventually artists like Ed Sheeran. Jack liked music too, but he was more of a one-song kind of kid. He'd find a song he liked, listen to it until we were all sick of it, and then pick a new song to kick around for a while. I am pretty sure he said the same thing about me, too.

I also tried ski club in middle school. It was fun, but racing down the slopes at Swiss Valley Ski Area in Jones, Michigan, was more Jack's style, not mine.

It was during these years that our differences became more apparent; yet our similarities formed a tighter bond among Jack, Justin and me (and later on, Matty).

Jack

You are only young once, and if
you work it right, once is enough.

- JOE E. LEWIS

My middle school years were a blast! I got to travel
to Canada to play in a hockey tournament with the
Irish Rovers, the travel team I made at the end of fifth
grade. Eventually, I was asked to play hockey at the
junior level, one skill level higher than the local travel
team I was on, but it meant a move to the Detroit area
(just me!) and Mom and Dad were not comfortable

with it. To be honest, I am really glad they said no. Deep down inside, I did not want to do it either. It would have been way too hard to leave my friends and family.

In elementary school we really did not have a legit art class; we had what was called Art Smart. It was basically a bunch of volunteers who would take turns coming in once a month and "teaching" a class. Beck was one of the Art Smart moms. I did secretly love it, even though I would roll my eyes when someone would teasingly say, "Jack, your mom is here today."

My creative juices really started flowing around middle school. My favorite class in middle school was art. I loved creating things, and how I could show my feelings through the art I created. I created pottery sculptures, drew and painted pictures, and carved. Really, I loved it all, and in middle school we had a real teacher for art!

I remember one summer I was invited by one of the art teachers to participate in a special summer program. The program involved using all different mediums of art and developing a niche or specialty. I thought long and hard about it – the opportunity to try more drawing, pottery, and photography piqued my interest. But in the end, I turned down the offer, and told my art teacher my answer would have to be "no" before I ever told Mom about the invitation. I knew my parents would want me to explore the opportunity – but seriously, during the summer? No way! That was my lake time! Besides, there were other ways to express my creativity. Doodling in class was one of them.

I stayed at the top of my class in middle school, but I had to work at it. Nick was just the opposite. He was super smart and barely had to apply himself. Although I have to admit, he was also quick to put his nose in a book to chill. I found other ways to chill – maybe because my definition of chill was me being in motion. That meant riding fast on the wakeboard behind the speed boat, or traipsing through fields while hunting for ducks, grouse, and pheasants with

Dad, Grandpa Larry, some of our cousins, and our German shorthaired pointer named Duke.

Now before I get my parents in trouble for using the "h-word" (hunting) I will say that my dad was always ALL about safety. Before we could even hold a BB or pellet gun, we took a gun safety course. Just like we took a boating safety course. If we were going to do something that required an adult-like understanding, like driving a boat or shooting a gun, there was always an official safety course with lots of follow-up lessons from Dad.

This was also the age when video games were all-consuming for most of my friends, and for Nick, too. I would occasionally hop on to play, but I preferred being outside, throwing a ball or slapping a puck on the ice. If I turned the TV on for anything good, it was usually a game or SportsCenter on ESPN for the latest sports news. I could sit down and watch any kind of game for hours – whatever was in season was my jam.

Nick liked sports too, but he loved his gaming time more. He was always switching back and forth between Xbox and PlayStation, and was the first in our family to figure out how to play online with other players – usually our cousins who lived a few towns over. Nick had an insane amount of focus for the things he loved, but for anything outside of his focus, he was like the "nutty professor." The obvious was less than obvious for that kid. Mom would ask him to go look for something, and he'd come back minutes later and swear he could not find it. So Mom would take a second look, and undoubtedly would find whatever it was, in plain view. We started calling this the "Nicky look" when Nick would miss things that were staring him in the face. Mom stopped asking him to look for things and started asking me.

I was always a "bigger is better" kind of kid, and my personality continued to grow during these years, when I realized I could make people laugh by being larger than life. Maybe I got that from my mom. We both love the largeness of life, but we expressed it in different ways. The attention was never on her, but she did love to make a big deal out of holidays and birthday parties. Our house was always the house for Christmas, always the place for the Fourth of July; and our parties and gatherings were often themed, thanks to Mom, Aunt Terri and their friends.

I loved Christmas! We would wake up, have breakfast, open presents – just the six of us – and then the rest of the family would come over after lunch for appetizers, more gifts, and a big family meal, followed by games and movies.

Sunday brunch was still a big deal for Mom. Whether we were home in Granger or at the lake house, we always had some kind of midmorning breakfast of pancakes, eggs, and bacon – if Nick could keep his fingers off the bacon long enough for the rest of us to grab a piece or two.

Big Mike, as we affectionately called our dad, started taking us to Chicago Blackhawks games when he was not out of town for work. Chicago was less than two hours away from our home in Granger, so we could be there and back in the same evening. Boy, were those fun times! We would go with our buddy Kevin and his dad; or with Nic, who was Nick's best friend. In fact, the four of us slept over at each other's houses so often, Mom started calling Nic's house "Camp Mensick."

In middle school, we got serious about riding dirt bikes up at the lake. Uncle Scott lived nearby, and he cut trails and cleared tracks on 20 acres in the woods at the edge of his property. He made sure to wear the track down before we arrived on weekends. We would ride for hours in the summer heat with Dad, Uncle Scott and our cousins, and then roast hot dogs on the grill or in the bonfire at night. That is still a family tradition. I loved the speed of racing our dirt bikes on the trails. Of course, Dad always tried to make us "drive cautiously," but I was always testing those rules and pushing my speedometer to the limit. I am pretty sure that Nick rode his dirt bike about three-quarters of the speed of mine. I was his threshold of speed. I cannot tell you how many times Nick would see me do a trick on my bike or take a big jump and tell me, "That is just stupid; you are going to get hurt!"

Nicknames were a big deal for us too – first at home, and then with our friends. We each had about 10 of them. I was Jacko, Jacks, Jacky, and Jacky Jack, just to name a few. And mom said I had a lot of "Jackisms" growing up – things only I could say to make everyone laugh. Like, one time I asked, "What is passtal code?!?" (Instead of "postal.") My dad thought it was funny stuff. And I could usually get a good laugh out of anyone who was listening (sometimes not even trying)!

Nicknames and special codes were my thing – they were **our** thing. Sometimes I did not even have to use full sentences when explaining a situation to my "bros" – my brothers and our friends. I just used one of our code phrases, gave them the raised eyebrow look, and they knew what I meant. I guess when you are really close to some people, you can kinda read their minds. We were quite the band of brothers – my real brothers and our friends.

THE GLORY YEARS
2011-2015

Nick

Youth is, after all, just a moment,
but it is the moment, the spark, that you
always carry in your heart.

- RAISA M. GORBACHEV

I was definitely living the dream in high school.
These were the glory years. Of course, I started out
shy and awkward. Who doesn't start out that way as
a freshman in high school? But I eventually grew out
of the awkward phase, and learned to embrace just

being shy. Jack and I both continued to get decent grades. And we both interned with Mrs. Campbell in the guidance office, and we both especially loved Mr. Dinatti, one of our gym teachers. We still had a blast doing things together, Jack and I, and we would swap stories about the moments that each other missed when we were apart.

We switched from playing travel hockey to playing for our high school team, the Penn High School Kingsmen. And we loved and respected our head coach. When we were not on the ice or with our team, Jack and I worked out together at FitStop, the local 24-hour gym in town. We had our routine. We'd go to school, stop home to change clothes, and head to the gym. Or come home, do some homework and chill, and then head to the gym late at night before bed. Either way, our hockey buddies would often meet us there. After our strength and conditioning workouts, we'd head home, make quick protein shakes, and take a shower. We went through phases where we tried to eat super-healthy. But I was a salty-snack kind of guy (I loved bacon, chips and my all-time favorite, Flamin' Hot Cheetos) and Jack always had a weak spot for sweets and carbs.

Our off-season workouts eventually rewarded us when we earned spots on Team Michiana – the local all-star hockey team. That was a shock for a kid who did not get a ton of ice time until halfway through his junior year. I was nominated as captain of Team Michiana for my senior year, and we won the big tournament championship. For the most part, Jack and I were known to be clean players out on the ice. But, we definitely stuck up for a teammate if there was an altercation or a flare-up. And Jack was known to settle a "situation" or two by getting between the players who were going at it.

We both still played the right wing position, although Jack filled in at center sometimes, too. Our high school team made it to the state championships my senior year, but we lost in the final round and took home the state runner-up crown. "Puck Dynasty" was our team theme that year. I received an All-State academic award as a student athlete and was voted Most Valuable Player on my team because I had the most points that season. That was a confidence-booster for me, as I started to realize that I was strong and steady, on and off the ice.

Both Jack and I worked at the Compton Family Ice Arena on the campus at the University of Notre Dame in South Bend, just a few minutes from our home. We figured, *why not get paid to be at the ice rink since we were always there anyway?* We worked in the Zamboni room, getting the rinks ready and cleaned up for the various skate sessions that took place every day. We were also skate guards for the open skate sessions, making sure everyone was skating in the right direction and sticking to the rink rules. We worked at a few of the learn-to-skate clinics too. When we were not out on the ice, we worked in the skate shop, handing out skate rentals, taking payments, checking on locker rooms, and answering questions. We were eventually trained to sharpen skates, which was convenient when our own skates needed to be sharpened.

We both also worked for an RV furniture company. Northern Indiana was home to a large percentage of the RV industry – in fact, that is how our dad made a living, working in RV sales. So there were plenty of short-term RV-related jobs around town.

With a little extra spending cash in our pockets, we grew an appetite for Taco Bell, Chipotle, Smoothie King, Dairy Queen, and snack shop stops at the local Speedway gas station. Since nicknames were already our thing, we were proud to be called the Bell Brothers, and actually increased our visits through the Taco Bell drive-thru so we could continue to live up to the nickname. It was totally normal for us to pull up and order 30 tacos at a time!

But we always shared our tacos with our friends; well, sometimes included among those friends was our dog! Heck, I even shared my Flamin' Hot Cheetos with Scout, our little Havanese puppy. He and I shared a special bond over those Cheetos. Scout was a rescue dog, and it was quite obvious that he came from an abusive home before he came to us. He would spend hours hiding under the furniture in our family room, but I could get him to come out from hiding with those hot Cheetos. Sharing was our thing, just as much as food was our thing.

We were the hangout house in high school for weekend hangs with our friends when we were not traveling for hockey or up at the lake with our family. Jack and I loved this because my mom would tend to buy more food if she knew friends were coming over; and also, because we could be lazy. Most of our crew was a mix of the old cul-de-sac gang and our teammates. We'd stay up all hours of the night playing ping pong and "sting pong." Mom and Dad were always on us for breaking the ping pong paddles. But truth be told, I think they were more than willing to replace the paddles if it meant that our house would continue to be the place to hang. As Justin and Matty got older, they would hang with us too.

I was still super shy, but I worked up the courage to ask Kacie to prom my junior year. She was a sophomore, but I did not care. She was the one I wanted to ask, and our friend Rachel kept bugging me until I did. I had arranged for Kacie to be excused from class one afternoon so I could ask her without a ton of other people around. Another friend took a guidance pass to her while she was in her biomedical science class, requesting that Kacie make her way down to the guidance office. But I met her in the hallway right outside her classroom with a big yellow sign I made the night before, and asked her to go to prom with me. A "promposal" was a bit weird for me and I was a bit awkward, but Kacie was so cute about it – and to top it all off, she said yes! So it was settled; we were going to prom together that year.

My senior year of high school was a blast. Outside of hockey, classes, and weekends at the lake, I made the most of my time hanging out with friends. I even took one of my best friends, Audrey, to the prom my senior year. Formal things like the prom were not really my thing. But I would be chill about it if it meant spending time with my friends. And that is what I remember most about that night, and graduation too. Not the formal dresses and tuxedos or caps and gowns, but the laughter and games and conversations with my crew, and with Jack, because they were his crew too.

My graduation party was up at the lake, just like every other special party we had that year. It was a joint party with my best friend from our senior class, Kevin Calhoun. We were both going to Indiana University that fall, so Mom had the party decked out with Penn High School and IU decorations. She even had mannequins made out of PVC pipe, dressed in red-and-white-striped pants and red IU T-shirts. Plastered on the face of the mannequins were fathead pictures of Kevin and me, and they were set out in front of the house to greet everyone as they arrived at the party. I think we played volleyball for three hours straight that night, with the sky lit up by the bonfire we built.

My love of music was ever growing and evolving throughout high school and college. I was happiest any time I was hanging out with the music cranking around my buddies, my brothers and our friends. And I started making memories and marking moments with special songs. "Riptide" by Vance Joy was our pontoon boat anthem. Ed Sheeran was always playing in the blue Jeep Cherokee that started out as mine and became Jack's when I left for Indiana University later that fall. During my freshman year of college, I was obsessed with "Cheerleader" by Jamaican singer OMI. My friends hated the song and gave me a ton of crap about listening to it, but honestly, I just did not even care. I marked seasons of my life with music, and that was how I stayed so chill.

Jack

It is not what you gather but
what you scatter that tells
the kind of life you've lived.

— HELEN WALTON

Ah, high school! I loved everything about these
years – the sweat, the pain, the growth, the glory, the
fun, the laughter, the late nights, the lakehouse and
the escapades. I lived for it all – especially for hockey.

It took a year or two for me to grow into my
high school body. During the summer between my

freshman and sophomore years, I went to Cedar Point amusement park with one of my best friends, Grant. I remember Grant's dad and his dad's friend Tom were riding all of the big roller coasters with us that day. While we were waiting in line for the biggest coaster in the park, we got to the height checkpoint in the line. And Tom asked the guy working the roller coaster to double-check my height, just to make sure I could ride the coaster. I laughed it off, thinking the request was just a sarcastic joke. But the park employee brought the height-checker-bar over to me, taking his job quite seriously. I didn't pass. **I didn't pass? What the heck?**

I could feel my face grow hot, and my eyes started to well with tears from embarrassment. Tom must have noticed the look on my face, because he burst into laughter and admitted that he stuck his foot under the bar when the employee looked up, so that the height-checker-bar would be taller than my head. A quick recheck **without** Tom's foot, and sure enough, I was tall enough to ride the coaster. But I was a bit self-conscious that I did not clear the height chart by more inches, with or without Tom's foot in the way. Thankfully, I shot up in height at the end of my sophomore year, and grew a few inches every year after that.

Just like all the other upperclassmen in South Bend, Mishawaka and Granger, the three neighboring cities in our community, Nick and I were familiar with all of the fast-food joints around town. But at some point, the Hana Yori hibachi bar became our thing. It was too pricey to be there on the regular, so the hibachi bar became the place we would go to celebrate birthdays and big moments with our family and friends. The steak and shrimp combo was my hibachi meal of choice. In fact, one of our best friends, Kevin, still has a picture on his phone of a hibachi chef making a fiery volcano out of onions.

I loved music, too, although I was not quite as obsessed as Nick. He made moments out of music, while I saw music as the soundtrack to the adventures of my life. I loved spontaneous playlists and listening to the radio for variety, but Nick could listen to the same dang song over and over again. And maybe he said the same thing about me, too. By my junior year of high school, I knew every word to every song by Kid Cudi and Juicy J. Just ask my friends. And as soon as Billy Joel's "Piano Man" came on the radio or over the stream, I was up on my feet, lip-syncing the words and playing the air piano along with the song. That was my gig – having fun, making people laugh, and enjoying the heck out of life.

YouTube videos became our thing in high school, and Nick and I would walk around quoting our favorite movie lines. Grant and I were known to sit together in class at the beginning of every school year, and by the end of the year, we would be moved away from each several times until we were finally on opposite sides of the classroom. We were definitely not the teacher's pets.

At some point in the middle of high school, I turned Grant into "Gurnt"– my favorite nickname for that guy. Everyone, and I mean **everyone** – including our friends and all of our friends' parents – called him Gurnt by the time we started our senior year of high school. Every time Nick or I passed him in the hallway at school, or out on the ice during practice, we would quietly call, "Guuuuurrrrnt!" It was just our thing.

Although there was one moment when I was not so certain about Grant being my friend. It was back in middle school. I had invited him for a sleepover at my house, and we were bouncing on the trampoline in his backyard. I had just gotten my very first phone earlier that day. I had **finally** convinced Mom and Dad I could be responsible with a phone now that I was "older and more mature." My exact words. It was the hottest phone on the market at the time – the Chocolate Touch. I was still in shock that my parents actually got it for me. Grant and I had the bright idea of tossing our phones on the trampoline to see how high they would go, but my phone hit one of the trampoline crossbeams and split in half. It was my fault, but I blamed it on Grant, because it was his dumb idea to toss our phones.

Without even thinking, I said, "Sh#! My mom is going to be so pissed at me." I was more concerned about ruining my reputation as being **responsible** than I was about my broken phone. *What would my parents say? Would they take it away and say I was not ready or mature enough?* I stormed off and left Grant outside. I know, real mature, right? No sleepover for us that night.

When I think about that time now, I know that must have been hard for Grant. He was an only child, and I knew he loved it when we included him in our brotherly banter. Like whenever I got mad at Nick, and knew I could get him back by mimicking his nervous stutter. Nick would respond by putting me in a headlock and throwing some pot shots at my arms and legs. Before we knew it, we were laughing and having fun again. And when Grant was around, he was in on the brotherly fun. The "bro banter."

Going to Chicago Blackhawks games with Nick, Justin, Matty and Big Mike (Dad) were some of my favorite family memories from those years. We loved watching Patrick Kane out on the ice, affectionately known in our house as Patty Kane. While playing street hockey, when one of us took a shot on goal, we would call it "hitting the top shelf where mom keeps the peanut butter." In the driveway, and out on the ice, we called each other and our teammates "Goon." It was just another one of those ridiculous nicknames.

After every hockey game, Nick and I would ride home in his blue Jeep Grand Cherokee and have real conversations about what we did well and what we could have done better in the game we just played. This was how we got better – by encouraging and challenging each other.

Before he retired, our high school hockey coach, Ryan Geist, told our parents we were leaders on the ice "who demonstrated what had to be done." He said that we each had a calming influence on the team and always wanted everyone to have fun, even though we were quiet out on the ice. Our physical trainer, Rick Freeman, was like a big brother to us. We were always goofing around and checking with him. That is just how we rolled. We always had each other's back, and that is what we told our teammates and our coaches, too. In fact, that was my motto during my senior season: "Always have your brother's back." We were a team and a brotherhood, for sure.

I took one of my best friends, Olivia, to prom in my senior year. She went to a boarding school just south of town, and her school did not have a prom. We got to know each other when her brother and I played travel hockey in middle school. Somewhere along the way, I told her I would take her to my senior prom. She knew a lot of my school friends, so it was not an awkward ask. And we had so much fun together that night, laughing and singing and dancing with each other and our friends.

My senior year, I was voted team captain at the beginning of the season by my teammates. I was fast and physical, and a leader on the team. I gave my best every time my blade hit the game ice. I skated hard to get back on defense just as much as I skated hard to score a goal.

We won the state championship that year, and Dad – aka Big Mike – got to give me my state championship plaque when we beat the Columbus Icemen in the 3A Indiana state championship finals. It was such a sweet victory after losing in an earlier round of state playoffs the season before, during Nick's senior year. I knew I had earned that championship – that **we** earned it as a team. I was still playing wing, although I missed Nick and his presence on the team.

GOING AWAY
School Year of 2014-15

CHAPTER 7

Nick

Freshman year of college was the best year of my life, especially with Kevin in Bloomington with me. It was just a three-hour drive from home. That meant we had the freedom to be our young-adult selves, and yet we were still close to the comforts of home. I am not going to lie – I missed home. I missed my parents, Mike and Becky; and my brothers, Jack and Justin and Matty; and I knew they all really missed me too. I checked in with Mom almost daily for her sake (and partly for mine, too), and with my brothers, to make sure they were staying in line. Not! To be honest, I missed hearing their voices and our brother bickering. Being away from them after all these years together was sometimes hard. I think my parents knew this because they would always answer the phone when I called and talk as long as I needed to talk.

During freshman orientation, Kevin and I found a favorite restaurant at the edge of campus called BuffaLouie's. It became our usual hangout spot and the place we went after football games in the fall. We even brought our parents there during parents weekend. When Kevin and I went home for school breaks that year, we'd drive the extra 30 minutes past home to catch our breath up at the lake. We carried on the tradition we'd made with the rest of the Savage brothers by stopping at the Shell gas station in Vandalia by the lake to grab snacks. We'd dig through our pockets and the crevices of our car cash and change to buy the basics – candy, chips and soda. We'd spent enough money at BuffaLouie's and in sneaking Pabst Blue Ribbon that year that the simple snacks were all we could afford.

There was a whole crew from the "574" at Indiana University that year (574 was our phone area code and it was the fastest way to explain the whole Granger-Mishawaka-South Bend area where we were all from). We had a group text called Blu City. The Blu was short for Bloomington. We were not all super close as a group in high school, but there was something about being three hours away from the same hometown that brought us together throughout the year. I met a ton of other new friends, too. The social scene was just like high school, but bigger and better. And the academics were challenging.

I could also sense a shift in my relationship with Mom and Dad that year, beginning at Thanksgiving when I came home for the first time during the fall semester. It seemed like we went from parents and their kids to peers. I was pretty sure Mom and Dad felt the shift, too.

I also rushed for a fraternity my first semester, but did not get a bid. I was super bummed about it, but I think Mom was glad because she kept saying something like, "Eighty percent of college students are not involved in Greek life and they are still having fun!" I did not completely buy it, but her reminder did make me feel better.

I decided not to rush during the spring semester of my freshman year, and that is when Mom showed her true colors. She said she was glad I decided not to do it, because sometimes fraternities and "nonsense" go hand in hand; my mom was always worried about the nonsense. I'm pretty sure I just shrugged my shoulders at her and said, "OK, Beck. OK," and then I let the fraternity idea slip away.

I started off my freshman year thinking I wanted to major in business, and then I did not really like it. And the truth was, I did not do as well as I thought I could in my courses. Mom made me take some kind of class that helps students decide on strengths and skills, etc., and it turned out that one of my skills was a love for chemistry. I knew what everyone was thinking: *Boring!* I know, right?! But in the second semester I dropped my business classes and signed up for chemistry and microbiology classes. And I did so much better. Go figure.

My first year away from home was really hard, and I could not wait to get home that summer. I loved college, but I was ready for a break. Jack and I were back working at the RV furniture job in Elkhart and picking up a few hours at the Compton Ice Arena together. And Jacky Jack was graduating from high school. I was kinda proud of that kid. He worked sorta hard for his diploma. Well, when he wanted to.

GRADUATION WEEK
2015

Nick and Jack

Jack

My graduation party was last weekend at the lake,
right after our actual graduation ceremony from
Penn High School. In fact, my cousin Grant and I
had a joint party at the lake. He graduated from the
same high school and was headed to IU Bloomington
(where Nick was) in the fall. By the time Grant and I
popped up to the lake for our joint party, the volleyball
net and our favorite game, bags, were already set up
for the festivities at the edge of the white party tent.

In usual Becky Savage fashion, the party was
themed! My mom does love her themes, so we

had Penn High School and Ball State University decorations, my favorite foods (including pulled pork), and pictures of me throughout the years. Of course, most of those pictures included Nick, too. All of the lake house crew, as well as our friends and family from town, were there. A bunch of my school friends and hockey teammates came up and spent the day with us, too. We goofed around on the pontoon boat, swam in the lake, caught some fish, and snuck a beer or two in the light of the bonfire. It was the best kind of party, with all of my favorite people. Mom always said our approach to special parties like that was to "go big or go home." And here we got to do both – go big and be at home.

The next weekend was a second weekend of parties, starting at my buddy Ryan's. Mom was coming with us to Ryan's party, and then we had plans to catch a few post-grad parties on our own. Just the guys. I was tired from a full day of work, itchy from a quick haircut, and giddy with excitement about the rest of the evening. I was seriously living the dream, and so grateful to have my bro Nick home from college and by my side. We were ready to roll.

Nick

Jack and I were together again. Man, I loved that kid. I was so proud of him. We had a blast celebrating him at the lake last weekend when the gang was together again, and it was just like old times. We had goofed around on the boat, went swimming and tubing, sung our favorite songs, and celebrated a new season by sneaking a few beers brought up to the lake by our friends – because we all knew Mom had her eye on the cooler, labeled "You Must Be 21!"

My freshman year of college and Jack's senior year of high school had flown by. And here we were – both headed to college. Justin, now affectionately called "Ju," was headed to college soon, too. Mom and Dad would have at least one year (or two, if I took extra time with those double majors) when their three oldest boys would be in college at the same time. Crazy.

But I did not have a ton of time to sit around thinking about it. Jack and I drove home from work in Elkhart that afternoon, blasting the music and stopping for quick haircuts along the way. I was not quite sure what I was going to wear that night, but I knew there was a bag of new shirts on my bed that Mom picked up last week before Jack's graduation. I would just grab one of those and be good with it. I knew I did not have to impress this crew, but I did like looking good every once in a while.

We took fast showers and headed out the door, driving my blue Jeep behind Mom's car, so we could leave our friend Ryan's graduation party at separate times if we had to. Dad, Ju and Matty were still up at the lake. They were more into fishing than attending another weekend of graduation parties, which was cool, because we knew all of our friends would eventually make their way up to the lake too as the summer wore on.

Looking back now, I wish we had all been together that evening – Dad, Ju, Matty, Jack and me – fishing and having a relaxed night without the drama that was about to unfold. I was simple and liked things easy, not out of order or difficult. I would have much preferred hanging out with a few friends than going to a big party with people I did not know. I probably would not have been faced with the peer pressure that led to the **One Choice** I wish I could take back. But hindsight is 20/20.

Jack

Most of the grad parties we visited tonight were just like the one Mom and Dad hosted for me at the lake house last weekend. That was such a great party! But something was off about the last party we went to tonight. It started out with just a few friends, but then an entire team of people showed up.

It was the place to be, because it was the party without parents that evening. I could tell Nick was uneasy the moment someone brought out the pills. Cups were filled, pills were passed. I do not even remember how or why I ended up with a pill. I just knew that the quickest way out of that situation was to take it and move on. Nick did the same thing, too. Then he was ready to go.

I was kind of hoping we could hang on for just a few more minutes. I wanted to finish my drink and say goodbye to a few of my friends who had just shown up. I made my way around the room, giving hugs and high-fives and "what-up bros," until a kid passed out and someone had to call 911. There were a few moments of chaos as some of the people at the party rushed to help the kid who passed out. The rest of us started to scatter.

I found Nick, the friend who drove us to the party, and the two other friends who had been hanging out with us that night. I knew my mom would be cool with them landing at our place that night. She's chill like that. I just hoped she would not see us come in, because we had been drinking and I did not want to get grounded. I knew she would probably still be up when we got home anyway. She was on the home stretch of writing her master's thesis and she was **always** up!

I loved my mom. Heck, my friends even loved my mom! But tonight, I wanted Beck to be upstairs so we did not get the questions!

Lady, running down to the riptide,

Taken away to the dark side,

I wanna be your left-hand man.

I love you when you're singing that song,

And I got a lump in my throat 'cause

you're gonna sing the words wrong.

- "RIPTIDE" BY VANCE JOY

THE GRAD PARTY
Saturday, June 13, 2015

Nick and Jack

Nick

There was some crazy stuff going on at the last grad party we visited for the night, and I was ready to get out of there. Jack seemed ready to leave, too. One kid passed out; I did not really understand what was happening. I just knew that everyone frantically started to scatter and it was time to go home.

We rode home quietly. No one really knew what to say. We were all a bit scared and wanted to put that party scene in the past. The further we drove from the party, the more relaxed we got. I heard someone let out a big sigh – probably Jack – and the friend who was driving us home that night cranked the radio. Ed Sheeran was on again. I loved Ed Sheeran. I found myself mouthing the words to the song, but inside my head, I wondered if we had made the best decision that night. The crowd, the drinking, the pills being passed around. The pills being passed around – what were we thinking? It was not sitting well with me.

We were dropped off around 12:30 a.m. that night, just under curfew like we had promised Mom a few hours earlier. Two of our friends asked if they could hang with us that night. One of the guys went to high school and college with me, and the other had been our teammate for the past few years. While we did not hang out with these guys as often as we hung out with our other friends, we had just spent the last few hours together visiting a bunch of grad parties. So, we decided it would be easier if we all just crashed at our house that night. We did not want Becky to worry about us. Plus, Jack had a thing about sleeping in his own bed.

We walked through the open garage door into the kitchen. I hit the garage door button on the way inside to close the door. That was the usual signal to say we were home – the sound of the electric door closing. Mom had left a light on in the kitchen for us. That was her usual signal to say, "Welcome home."

My mom leaned over the second-floor balcony to say, "Hey guys, I am going to bed soon. Don't stay up too late." She paused and then said, "I mean it. We have stuff to do tomorrow!" I know she was just making sure we were both home, and that we were not drunk. Thank God we were not drunk – but the thought of those pills we took still bothered me.

"All right, we are grabbing a snack and heading to bed," I said.

And then I did what I would always do when I wanted to push away any kind of doubt or regret – I grabbed some food. Beck always said I was a little bit of a "carb-fiend." Give me all the carbs and I'll be happy forever – crackers, bread, pizza, cake, and especially bagels. Plain bagels with cream cheese.

And I liked the **real** kind of bagels, made fresh, from the local grocery store. They were my easy go-to, and the kind of stuff Mom always kept on hand. In fact, I had been looking forward to having a bagel all night.

I knew Mom had gone to the grocery store after Ryan's graduation party. Jack and I had popped home at one point to grab some food, and Mom had just pulled up with a car full of groceries. We helped her unload the groceries, carrying the bags into the kitchen. I grabbed the deli meat and Hawaiian bread from the bags while she was trying to sort through everything and put it away. We stuffed our mouths full – me with a turkey sandwich and Jack with a bunch of grapes – and we gave her a quick hug before we dashed out again. "Love you, Beck!" we shouted. She had kindly offered to give us a ride for the rest of our night out on the town, but we were riding with my friends, and we hopped in their car.

Now back at home again after a night of partying, I pulled the bagels out of the pantry and Jack grabbed the cream cheese from the fridge. Tonight was a treat, because Mom had bought a fresh tub of whipped cream cheese, which she only picked up on special occasions. We moved around the kitchen, bumping into each other, and talking over each other about the party we were just at. The last party was not our usual crowd, but it was "the place" to land after visiting a couple of more formal grad parties, and it was the parent-free party of the night.

Beneath the casual conversation in our kitchen, we all knew that Jack and I had tried oxy at the party after downing a few beers, but no one talked about it. While we were still carb-loading with bagels and getting sleepy, we received a text from a friend who had just left the party.

It was now 1 a.m. The friend asked if we were feeling OK, because he said another guy who took a few pills at the party had just been whisked away in the ambulance after having been resuscitated. He even used the word "overdose" in his text. Dread and fear dropped hard in the pit of my stomach. I was not feeling well, but I reasoned with myself that it was the dread and fear making me sick, not the oxycodone in my system. We should not have been there. We should not have taken those pills. And I wanted nothing to do with that kind of party scene ever again. That was not even really my crowd.

Jack

I was tired, but feeling a little buzzed from a night of partying with my friends. It felt so good to be done with high school, and I could not wait to get to Ball State in a few months. My muscles were still sore from moving RV furniture in and out of storage that morning. And my neck was still scratchy from a few stray hairs that were stuck to my skin after this afternoon's haircut. I smelled like a mix of sweat, polyester (from my brand-new golf polo), a touch of sporty deodorant, and a splash of beer. Or maybe that was my breath. Anyway, I was ready to take a shower and crash for the night – after a few bagels.

Bagels were our thing, Nick and me. Our younger brothers, Justin and Matt, liked bagels too, but they were at the lake house for the weekend fishing with my dad, so this bag was all ours. I was hoping that the bagels would settle the upset feeling I was starting to have in the pit of my stomach. I had less than two beers at the party, so I did not think that was the issue. But maybe it was the combination of a hot evening, the party-hopping, and end-of-school-year exhaustion that was finally catching up to me.

Or maybe it was the pill. But I did not want to think about the pill. I was just glad that everything was cool now. I still do not know why we said yes to taking those pills. But it was something Nick and I did together, and now we could put it behind us together, too.

"Hey Nick, I am out. I cannot stay awake, dude. I need to head to bed. See you in the morning, bro. 'Night, guys."

Through Jack's Eyes

Every day may not be a good day,
but there is good in every day.

— UNKNOWN

Sunday, June 14, 1:00 a.m.

On my way up to my bedroom that night, I brushed past the picture frames Mom had on display on a table in the foyer. In doing so, I accidentally bumped into one of the frames, knocking it over onto the floor. I watched the frame tumble to the ground like it was all happening in slow motion, certain the glass would break. I winced, moved my bare feet out of the way, and put my hands to my ears as if covering my ears would muffle the sound so it would not wake or startle Mom. Nothing broke, thank God. I felt the sick pit in my stomach growing as I picked up the picture frame and placed it back on the table. It was a picture of me and Nick when we were little. God, I loved that guy. He was my brother – my bro – and one of my best friends.

Eighteen months and three days. That is how long my big bro Nick has been breathing without me around. He's a Thanksgiving baby, born on November 28, 1995, and I showed up a year and a half later on May 25, 1997. Nick's a handsome guy; I am not going to lie. Those long, tan legs, the blonde hair, the blue eyes, the 6-foot-1-inch frame. You get the picture. Between the two of us, Nick is known as the quiet one. And me, I guess I am known as the adventurous one. That is what happens when you are brothers close in age and separated by only one year in school. It is also what happens when you share the same friends, teammates, and teachers.

It is the classic sibling comparison. Nick is quiet, I am loud. Nick is steady, I am impulsive. Nick is shy, I am more outgoing. Nick is calm, and I tend to get more excited about things. Beck says I am a firecracker. But the truth is, I had to find some way to match Nick's strength and keep up with his steady, calm presence, so it seemed only natural to be a little larger than life at times. But still in a chill way.

This past year was a big adjustment for me with Nick away at college. I went to visit him and his friends a few times at IU in Bloomington. But I was looking forward to more trips back and forth between Bloomington and Muncie in the coming fall, when I would be at Ball State and he returned to Indiana University. Even so, he made it clear that the fall semester was going to be a hard one, with his double major in chemistry and microbiology. I did not know how he was doing a double major in two hard subjects, but he always made school look so easy.

Nick was not just my big bro – he was also my role model, my teammate, and like I said before, one of my best friends. We had done almost **everything** together our entire lives, from school to sports to neighborhood hangouts. We played hockey together, rode dirt bikes together, went tubing and wake surfing off the boat together, worked summer jobs together. Heck, we even interned in the high school guidance office together. So it was totally normal that Nick would spend the night hanging out with me and my friends as we hopped between grad parties for a second weekend in a row. They were his teammates and friends, too.

Man, I was so tired, and still not feeling so great, but I could not crash without taking a shower. That was just my thing. I grabbed a clean pair of underwear from the pile on my floor, and walked down the hall to the bathroom across from Nick's room to take a quick shower.

CHAPTER 10

I glanced into Nick's room as I opened the bathroom door directly across the hallway. The hall light was still on, casting a shadow of light into his room, and I could see his University of Michigan banner still hanging in the middle of the wall. I thought that sharing a college dorm with a roommate would change the way Nick settled back into living at home that summer, but nothing had changed. Clothes were scattered in piles on the floor. Books were tightly stacked to fill every inch of the bookcase by his bed. And the covers on his bed were still pulled back from our early wake-up call so we could be at work that morning in Elkhart, a good 20-minute drive from home. Who knows how long that glass of water had been on his nightstand? But it was always there. I had one in my room, too.

For as much as Nick loved to spend time reading or chilling in his room, he was also the kind of kid who could crash anywhere. We'd wake up sometimes to find him sleeping in the living room, or on the sofa in the basement. Mom would tease him, saying he was too lazy to get up and walk up to his room.

Tonight, he was not being lazy, he was just being kind. He knew I would want to crash in my bed, so without even saying anything to me, he told our buddies that they would crash with him in the basement. When we were not raiding the fridge in the kitchen, or watching a game with the rest of the family in the living room, the basement was our usual hangout spot. It was where we played games with our friends and turned the traditional game of ping pong into "sting pong." This version of the game was a guys-only kind of game, because it meant taking off our shirts and seeing how hard we could pelt each other with the ping pong ball. We played until our forearms got tired, or until one of us could not take the stinging shots anymore.

I paused as I reached for the shower nozzle to turn the water on. Did I hear those guys playing ping pong in the basement? Nah, it was too late for a game, and they had looked just as tired as I did when we turned out the kitchen lights to head to bed. It must have been my imagination playing with me. That weird feeling in my belly kept getting worse. *Am I getting sick?* But this was a new kind of feeling for me. Not the way I felt other times I got sick. I knew this shower needed to be quick.

I barely felt the warm water running down over my head. But I did feel thirsty – so thirsty that I could not wait to chug a few gulps of water from the glass on my nightstand as soon as I got back to my room. Who knows how long the glass had been sitting there, or even if the glass was mine or Justin's? I did not care. Justin was at the lake house with Dad, so he would never notice even if it was his. And I was just so tired, and dizzy. The dizziness was coming on fast and hard. I fumbled for a towel, dried off, slid on the clean pair of underwear, made my way down the hall to my room, took a big gulp of water, and crashed hard in my bed.

CHAPTER 11

Through Nick's Eyes

Let your smile change the world, but
do not let the world change your smile.

- UNKNOWN

Sunday, June 14, 1:00 a.m.

Jacky Jack. I watched him knock over the picture frame in the hallway and wait for it to crash. Even though I had just turned off the kitchen light, I could see the relief on his face when he picked up the frame and it was still in one piece. Whew! I was relieved for him too.

"Come on, guys," I said to the two friends who decided to hang out at our place that night.

"We're sleeping down here."

As I started down the steps to the basement, I heard Jack walk up the stairs, pause for a moment in his room, and walk down the hallway. *He must be taking a shower.* I was too tired for that, but I knew his routine better than anyone else. As close as we were, we never shared a room. It was always Jack and Justin sharing a room. But my room was right across from the bathroom, and I knew that a nighttime shower was his thing.

One of my buddies took the floor, and the other buddy and I crashed on the L-shaped sofa with our feet almost touching in the corner. We were all so tired; we barely talked as we drifted off to sleep. I might have fallen asleep faster, except for that sick feeling in my stomach. I knew everything would be all right as soon as I got some sleep. As I lay there, drifting off to sleep, I thought of Jack. I could not believe my little bro was finished with high school already. His senior year went so fast.

And what a year it was; I am so proud of that kid. The way he stepped up as hockey team captain and led the team to the state championship; the way he took over my guidance office intern role and made it his own. While I loved giving new students a tour of our high school, Jack did not think twice about answering the annoying office phones or handling difficult questions from disgruntled parents and students.

Although he wasn't afraid of leading and taking responsibility, he also liked to have fun and goof off. He was a daredevil, always taking our tricks, challenges and dares to the next level. Take, for instance, the time Mom and Dad left us with Grandma at the lake house. Mom had gone back to work full-time that year, so Grandma came up to the house to stay with us during the day while Mom and Dad were at work. They said, "No dirt bikes while we're gone." And as soon as they left, Jack convinced me there was no harm in taking a quick little ride while Grandma was busy in the kitchen. We would be out and back before anyone knew we were gone, and before Mom and Dad would get home.

Sitting proud on his dirt bike that afternoon, Jack took the long and high approach to speed bumps on the track, but luck was not in his favor that day. He got a little twisted during a jump, landed wrong, and crashed into a tree at the edge of the homemade racetrack we built with Dad and a few buddies a few years earlier. Jack laid on the ground moaning and wincing in pain, but refusing to cry. No doubt he heard Mom's voice in his head, "Do not come crying unless there is blood." You could take Mom out of the nurse, but you could never take the nurse out of Mom.

(I yawn as drowsiness begins to take a hold of me)

I dropped my bike and ran over to help him up off the ground. I knew in an instant that something was wrong with his shoulder. We walked our bikes back to the house, carefully and slowly. Jack muscled his way through the one-handed steering with his bike. After we walked inside, Grandma glanced up to see Jack sit down calmly on the sofa. He whispered to me, "Go get me some Tylenol," and I went to the bathroom to see what Mom had in the medicine cabinet to help with his pain.

Grandma figured we had been up to something. When she pressed us with questions, we spilled the beans because of Jack's increasing pain. Dad just pulled up as Grandma was beginning to figure out what was going on, and next thing I knew, Jack was in the car and headed to the hospital back in town. Mom met Jack and Dad at the emergency room. Within a few minutes, the doctors told us that Jack had a compound fracture in his collarbone – one that would require surgery later that day. Later, while Jack was in the final weeks of healing from his collarbone injury, he was out trying tricks and flips on his Razor scooter and fell and broke his thumb. That kid was used to chaos.

But he always had a smile. And not just any smile. It was a semi-crooked, smirk kind of smile. It sounds goofy, but it actually made him quite popular with the ladies. With his crooked-smirk-smile, the tousled brown hair, those green eyes, and his medium, always-fit frame, Jack had enough charm to light up a room. He was one of a kind. Just ask our friends — they would say so, too.

And he was a natural at everything he tried, especially in sports. I had to work to be good at stuff, but Jack – well, Jack was just **good.** And he had enough confidence for both of us. Even when he poked fun at me hard, I could not stay mad for long. Conversation came easy for him, while I got nervous and often stuttered when I was around a pretty girl. If Jack noticed, he would punch me in the arm and say, "Niccccc, Nicccccc, Niccccolodeon!"

We shared a ton of friends. That is what happens when you are 18 months apart. And Jack loved spending time with every single one of those friends, often in large groups. I loved our friends too, but I was a little more shy, and recharged best when I was with just one or two of our friends. Plus, we loved to spend time with our two younger brothers, too.

Justin turned 16 this year and just finished his sophomore year in high school. And Matty turned 11 and just finished fifth grade. He was getting ready for middle school. We all used to say he was "the last of the Mohicans," a phrase made popular by a movie with the same title. It was part of our brotherly banter. Gosh, we love those little bros. And they love us too. I could see it in the way they watched us from behind the ice rink glass at our games; the way Justin and his friends did some of the same things we liked to do, and the way Matty watched us wistfully from the dock at the lake while we goofed around on the boat out on the water.

Sometimes I wondered how Mom and Dad did it all – how they made life so simple and fun and carefree for the four of us. How they easily floated between the lake house and home, how they bent and flexed around our plans, how they were either behind the bench or in the stands for every one of our hockey games. They made the best memories for us. Like when we were little and Dad would be out of town for work, so Mom would take us to McDonald's PlayPlace until Jack, Justin and I were worn out and sweaty. Sometimes we'd meet other friends there, too. Then she'd round us up, and buy a small treat or ice cream cone for each of us before she strapped us back in our car seats and headed home for showers, books and bedtime. As silly as this may sound, I smile everytime I pass a McDonald's, thinking of these times.

And the truth is, I kind of missed Mom and Dad when I was away at college this year. And I know Jack will too. I checked in with Mom almost every day. I loved to picture Mom's smile when she answered the phone and heard me say, "What-up, Beck?" or "Beckyyyyyyyyy!" Ah, that was so much fun! So, a word to the wise for all of my little brothers when they go off to college: **call Mom.**

This is where Jack and Nick's story ends,
but it is not the end of our story.

CHAPTER 12

Through Becky's Eyes

You were my greatest hello, my saddest goodbye, and the biggest 'what if' I will question for the rest of my life.

- STEPHANIE BENNETT-HENRY

Sunday, June 14th began like all my other Sundays – with laundry. Having four active boys in a family of six, there was always plenty of dirty clothes. My Sunday morning laundry pickups usually started in my own room before I swooped into the boys' rooms to pick up their dirty clothes. I gave the boys responsibility with other household chores, except for this one.

It was the one chore I did for my boys. But I expected them to put their clean, folded clothes away in their dressers and closet drawers. Nick thought it was much easier just to pull clean clothes straight from the pile, so he always left his clothes on the floor. I did not make a big fuss over it.

I was up early that morning to finish an assignment for a class. The Zac Brown Band had just come out with a new album and I was obsessed with "You Make Loving You Easy." So, that song was playing loudly – I mean really loudly! It was Momma's way of saying "Time to get up, boys." The song reminded me so much of my boys – they were so easy to love.

Jack's room, which he shared with his brother Justin, was at the end of the hallway. I walked into his room to pick up their laundry. Looking at Jack, I thought, *He looks just like an angel.* Little did I know the truth of that thought on that morning. The longer I watched him sleep, the more worried I became, because I could not see his chest moving. I know it is not normal to watch your children breathe . . . but when you are a nurse, that is what you do.

I walked over to his bed and shook him – nothing. I started to yell his name, "JACK! JACK!!!" Nothing. I rubbed his sternum – this is something that medical people do when they are trying to arouse someone – again, nothing. I felt for a pulse, and this sick feeling came over me. I could not find his pulse . . . *Am I in the right spot . . . this is not happening . . . what is going on?!* I left Jack and ran downstairs to get my cell phone to call 911. I yelled for Nick as I ran back upstairs. I really wanted someone to come and help me. I still could not comprehend what was going on. I just wanted help.

I returned to Jack's room with the 911 operator on the phone. She kept trying to tell me how to do CPR. I kept telling her that I knew how. "Just please get me help." It was really a no-win situation for both of us.

I picked Jack up out of his bed and began CPR. It was one of the worst moments of my life. I continued to yell for Nick to come and help me. One of Nick and Jack's friends came up from the basement. I looked at him and he looked just as distraught as I felt. He was upset and crying. "What can I do to help?" he asked. I said, "I really do not know what is going on. Please, please, please, I need help!" He asked what he could do, and I told him to go find someone to help me. I know it was just a matter of minutes, but it truly did feel like an eternity.

I heard sirens, and when I looked up there were people there. They took over the resuscitation attempts on Jack. They asked me what was going on, and I told them, "I have no idea." I was frantic. Jack was in bad shape, and I had no idea what was going on in my house.

I walked to my bedroom while they worked on Jack, and that is when Nick's friend once again appeared. I remember looking at him and yelling, "What is going on in my house??"

That is when he told me, "They tried Oxy last night!"

"Wait, what?! They did WHAT?"

"They tried Oxy at the party last night."

"Oh my God, where is Nick?"

I turned to the paramedics and I screamed that Jack needed Narcan (the medication designed to reverse the effects of opioid overdose).

I thought, *Where is Nick? Why is he not coming to help?*

It was then that I noticed a paramedic leaving Jack's side and heading down the stairs to my basement. I asked him, "Where are you going? Why are you leaving Jack?"

He kept walking . . .

I was a mess.

A few minutes later the same paramedic came up from my basement and called for a coroner. Again, I thought, *What is going on in my house?*

The police arrived.

I was crying.

I was confused.

I was in shock.

The police officer told me that there had been a second 911 call. The boy's friends had called 911 from the basement because they needed help with Nick.

My boys.

They were gone.

Mike, their dad – I needed to reach him at the lake house.

I called. I could not get him.

I called the neighbors to tell him to come home immediately.

I told them there had been an emergency.

Friends, family members and neighbors started to show up, asking what they could do. The local news media showed up, too. My friend Maureen took care of making sure the reporters stayed out of the house to give all of us some privacy. It was a long day for them, and a horrific day for us.

I could not bring myself to go to the basement and see Nick. I was in shock. I was scared. I was in so much pain.

I did not want to leave the house until my boys left. But when that moment came, I ushered everyone onto the back deck, so they would not have to watch as the paramedics and the coroner took my boys' lifeless bodies in bags from the house. I did not want that to be my last image of my sweet boys.

Later that day, when Justin and Matt showed up at the house, Justin immediately went to the bedroom he and Jack shared. He laid on the floor, and cried and cried. Justin and Jack had shared a special brother bond. When Justin, or "Ju" as we called him, was little, Jack would crawl into Justin's crib to steal some of his pacifiers – which he called "tacis" – and then fall asleep next to him, still hoarding his pacifiers in his tiny hands. When we moved into our Woodington Court house at the beginning of elementary school for them, Justin and Jack wanted to share a room. They had been sharing a room for almost 15 years. So, that day in June, Justin did not just lose his older brothers, he lost his roommate, and a part of himself too.

A month later, toxicology test results confirmed that a mixture of hydrocodone – a prescription painkiller – and alcohol were what killed my boys. Their deaths were ruled accidental by the St. Joseph County Deputy Coroner's Office, but some questions about the circumstances leading up to their overdoses still remain unanswered.

RIPTIDES AND REFLECTIONS

How Our Choices
Change Our Lives

Everything you do is based on
the choices you make. It is not
your parents, your past relationships,
your job, the economy, the weather, an
argument or your age that is to blame.
You and only you are responsible for every
decision and choice you make. Period.

– POWER OF POSITIVITY

CHAPTER 13

Becky

Nick and Jack passed away in the early morning hours of Sunday, June 14th. That night, the four of us who were left slept at the lake house. In fact, we never slept in our Granger house again. We just could not. There were too many memories of those final moments for me, and too much of a void for the rest of the family. Just a short 30-minute drive away, our house at Donnell Lake in Michigan became our full-time home that summer. Our friends and family rallied around us following the deaths. They had our house cleaned out and ready to put on the real estate market within weeks. They helped us make plans for the funeral service at the church that we attended in South Bend. And they fed our family for four months straight that summer – driving up to the lake with meals they made.

Four days after that fatal morning, hundreds of people showed up at the viewing to pay their respects: our extended family, friends, Nick and Jack's teachers, coaches, teammates, fellow hockey players, and people from the community. The boys were the big story in town. Hundreds of people came to offer their condolences. Many people generously donated to the memorial fund in Nick and Jack's names – a fund we would later use to start a foundation.

Matty designed and ordered bracelets the day before the viewing as a way to process his own grief. The bracelets said "Nick/Jack #SavageStrong" on the outside and "Forever in our hearts" on the inside. I was upset when I realized that Matty was selling the bracelets at the funeral instead of just passing them out.

"Matt, are you **selling** these bracelets to people here at the viewing?" I was horrified. But I could not stay mad at his response.

"Mom, we're going to use this money to do something good in Nick and Jack's name." Our 11-year-old son already knew what needed to be done in order for us to survive this tragedy – **do something good in Nick and Jack's name.**

The following day, we said our final goodbyes. To be honest, I do not remember much from that day. The boys' hockey coaches talked about the brothers' character and how they had left an impact on all of the other players. The minister talked about the day Nick and Jack were confirmed, and read their statements of faith. I do remember feeling an overwhelming sense of joy filling my heart as I listened to their testimony of faith.

There is not much more in my memory from that day except one other thing. On the way to our church, the song "See You Again" by Wiz Khalifa came on the radio and it really spoke to my heart.

I will see them again someday. I felt that the song played for a reason – I needed to hear it. At that moment, I decided that others needed to hear it too. So, at the last minute, we decided to have that song play as the boys left the church in the caskets carried by their brothers, family and friends. To this day, everytime I hear the song, I think of Nick and Jack.

Back at the lake house that summer, we grieved privately and began to piece our lives back together. Mike, Justin, Matty and I were now a family of four, taking care of each other at the lake house and looking online for a new home in time for the start of school that fall. Matt and Justin would stay at the same school where the older boys had graduated – Penn High School. They would play on the same hockey teams and spend time with some of the same friends, or the younger siblings of Nick and Jack's friends.

We moved on, but painfully and slowly. We also moved on cautiously. I continued the Momtalks I had given to Nick and Jack with Justin and Matt, but this time the talks were not just about illicit drugs, drinking and driving, and sex. They were about prescription drugs – opioids – too.

We started a foundation in Nick and Jack's memory, focused on primary prevention – to promote awareness and education on the dangers of prescription drug misuse and abuse. If my boys could make one uneducated choice, and take a pill at a party, so can thousands of other young people. Perhaps if my boys had heard about these dangers in an auditorium or gymnasium full of peers and friends – like the assemblies I speak at now – they would have made a different choice on that night in June.

There is a huge stigma to erase when it comes to the topic of overdosing, and about who it can happen to. It does not just happen to "narcs," or addicts, or people who regularly misuse and abuse drugs. It also happens to first-time users like Nick and Jack.

Accidental overdosing – or any kind of overdose, for that matter – is like a riptide. Riptides are powerful currents of ocean water flowing away from the shoreline, perpendicular to the beach, and back out to sea. These currents are also known as "killer currents" because they are hard to recognize, and can swiftly carry a person out to sea in a narrow jet of water. If you have ever been caught in a riptide or a rip current before, then you know that the natural reaction is to swim against the current and back to shore. But the riptide is almost always too strong to fight – especially if you are swimming against it – and being caught in one can easily lead to drowning. In fact, according to the U.S. Lifeguarding Association, more than 80 percent of annual lifeguarding rescues are related to someone being caught in a riptide current. If you've ever felt that kind of riptide, you know how strong and fast the force is. It is there before you even know it, and once you are in it, it is hard to get out of it.

That is how it must have felt that night after Nick and Jack took those pills. Their accidental overdose was the riptide of one mistake, the one moment of peer pressure, the *One Choice* that carried them away. And it can carry you away too, if you are not aware of the dangers.

One Choice can have a painful ripple effect. The riptide of the choice that Nick and Jack made to take someone else's prescription pills while under the influence of alcohol has rocked our lives, and the lives of our friends and all of their families too. Even Tucker, our family dog, felt the effects of the boys' absence. They loved that dog. And now he is my shadow, knowing I need his love and comfort while I do the hard work of carrying on our sons' legacy. Everyone who loved Nick and Jack has a lifetime sentence of grief caused by their passing. Never in a million years could the boys have imagined the ripple effect caused by their *One Choice.*

Nick and Jack both had big dreams to graduate from college, have careers, travel to fun places, grow up with their friends, get married, have their own families, enjoy their very own lake houses with pontoon boats, coach their kids someday, and make their own spring break memories. Those dreams also died that night.

Now we celebrate Christmas and go on spring break as a family of four. We think about how every event would be different if Nick and Jack were still there. But they are not. Their friends get together to celebrate birthdays, and wish that Nick and Jack were there. But they are not. We are so thankful that we have been wrapped in love and support from our community; and yet, nothing is a substitute for the presence of my boys.

In a video we created to show at my presentations at school, Mike begs for 10 more seconds with our boys. If only we had 10 more seconds; 10 more seconds to give big hugs and tell our boys we love them, 10 more seconds for them to make a different choice – to make a **better** choice – so that the ripple would not leave such a hole in our lives.

So let Nick and Jack – and their fatal choice – be a lesson to you, so that you make positive choices as you keep on living.

FOR THE BOYS

Letters, With Love

I have not heard your voice in years, but my heart has conversations with you everyday.

- J.N.

"For the boys" was the phrase most commonly used when people donated to the memorial fund or did good deeds in Nick and Jack's name. It was also why Mike and I started a foundation. And it is why a ton of the boys' friends still participate in random acts of kindness every year on Jack's birthday, May 25 (5/25) – also known around town as

"525 Day" (the same numbers as their hockey jerseys and their foundation).

A friend of theirs still loves to show up at the local McDonald's just to buy 10 ice cream sundaes and pass them out to guests. Everytime he does it, he posts a picture on social media under the hashtag #525day. These are examples of how a bunch of people started doing something good "for the boys" around town.

In the past six years, since we laid the boys to rest, I have asked a few of their closest friends to share some fun stories and memories to honor Nick and Jack's memory, **for the boys.** Here are those letters.

A letter we received at the funeral, June 2015

Sophie was a dear friend of both Nick and Jack. She started hanging out with their circle of friends when her brother, Michael, started playing hockey with the boys.

Dear Mr. and Mrs. Savage,

Since before my time in high school I always knew who the Savage brothers were, because I have heard about them from countless people. Little did I know how much of an impact the two boys and their family would have on me, my family, my friends, and my high school memories. My freshman year was dominated by hockey games. I never mentioned the Penn hockey team without hearing Nick or Jack Savage. They were practically identical brothers.

Not much later, I had the pleasure of meeting and befriending one of the boys' really good friends, Olivia – who only had good things to say about the Savage brothers. She was one of Jack's best friends – period. I remember my sophomore year when one of my best friends went to prom with Nick. I was very jealous when she invited me over to see them get pictures taken. I insisted on being in between the two of them for all their pictures – sorry.

I also recall during my sophomore year how Nic raved about his best friend, Nick Savage. I had no idea the extent to which the boys had spread themselves – they knew everyone! I remember when I met their cousin Grant, thinking to myself, If Grant is so nice, then it must mean Nick and Jack come from a nice family. *They really did. It was always a good night when both brothers scored. Whenever that happened, I always turned to find Mr. and Mrs. Savage and they would be cheering.*

Thanks to Nick and Jack, I was introduced to so many people. I was given the opportunity to connect with so many people. It is impossible for me to forget Jack's senior season. He was easily the most valuable player. It was exciting to see him on the ice. I told Casey one time before a game, "We are going to win. It will be close, but I just know Jack will score." And he did. The state championship game easily stood out in Jack's career, and I am so glad that I saw it. I remember the ride home. Everyone was talking about the game and Jack belted out a country song and "Riptide."

My first time at the Savage house was the same night my brother Michael scored his first Penn hockey goal. It meant so much to my family and me. I figured that it would not matter to anybody else, but I was surprised and thrilled when Jack said to me, "Michael had a good game tonight and a really good goal." It really is the littlest things.

I am so, so, so sorry that Jack and Nick left this world. They were both beyond fantastic boys. And my times with them, though few, mean a lot to me. Jack and Nick are navigating the next phase together and they will continue to look out for each other, as well as those left behind. I will not ever forget them. And I'll be sure to tell their story over and over again. Jack hugged me on the night of June 13, after having said, "Hey Sophie." I am so, so glad to have gotten to know him to that point – a hug! He and Nick were so funny and I will never look at a blue Jeep again without thinking of them. The Savage family is so strong and loved. What an impact they made in such a short time.

Love, Sophie

June 2020

Kevin was their school friend and shared his freshman year at Indiana University with Nick.

Dear Nick and Jack,

It has now been over five years since we've been together. For me, the reality of living a life without you in it is something that will take a bit longer than that to settle into. Five years is a long time and I am starting to miss things that I realize I no longer have, now more than ever.

I miss those late nights on the lake, talking for hours. I miss those dap-me-up handshakes. I miss those times on the bench when you laughed during serious situations. I miss the way we made fun of each other. I miss your positivity and insanely relaxed outlook on life. I miss your confidence that used to rub off on me. Most of all, I miss taking on life with you by my side.

Despite the fact I may not be able to continue making memories with you, I know you've been looking after me from heaven and are proud of the person I have become since you left. I feel your presence in my everyday life and know that you have helped guide me to real happiness. With your help, I graduated college, found my way into a career I like, moved across the country, found that girl I was always looking for, and became someone I am proud to be. I wish you were here to see it.

Not a day goes by that I do not think about you. Thank you for looking after us and being angels for everyone who loves you. We love you like crazy.

Your friend,

Kevin

June 2020

Jameson, also known as "Jay," is an older cousin to Nick, Jack, Justin and Matthew. Jay was like an older brother to Nick and Jack. He is one of their oldest friends, and most likely their very first friend when they were little.

Dear Nick and Jack,

It has been five years since you passed and not a day goes by that I do not think about you two goons. A lot has happened since we last talked. Marie and I bought a house in 2016 and have been working on making it our home ever since. We got married in May 2017 and the wedding was a blast. Justin was in the wedding party, and did a good job bringing some life to the party. You taught him well. Having the family together reminded us of what is so special about us Savages.

I started racing in 2016, which has been a lot of fun. Holly has also started racing now, and from the sounds of it, Matthew and Peter are not far behind. Grandpa finally "finished" the Lotus and has been working on getting the bugs worked out of the car. Exciting times are ahead, as we have the potential to have six Savages on the track at the same time within the next few years. Talk about chaos. I cherish the memories I have with you guys coming to Road America for the runoffs. I specifically cherish the road trips there, picking you guys up from your house at midnight and driving through the night, so we were the first ones through the gate in the morning. Or sleeping in a tiny tent while it was 40 degrees and pouring rain outside. Either way, it did not matter, we were at the racetrack!

I miss the first couple of years we had duck hunting together. Whether it was trying to find our way to the spot in the dark, or driving around in the afternoon looking for good spots to set up the next day while listening to "Boys 'Round Here" on repeat. I will never forget the first outing on Donnell Lake where Nick shot better than all of us even though he was the least "experienced." That grin on his face, forever captured in the picture of the four of us next to the boat with geese in our hands. Last year Matthew and I went duck hunting on opening day and Matthew got his first wood duck! He was ecstatic, so much so that he decided to take a nap in the boat next to the heater. That was the only bird we saw all day, but it was still fun to be out on the water with your brother. Every year, the foundation your mom and dad started holds a "525 Hunt" at Rolling Hills Preserve, where we gather a bunch of close friends and family to *go hunt pheasants for the day. I try to make it down each year and usually hunt with Grandpa. Just like we used to years ago on Thanksgiving.*

Until we meet again.

Love, Jay

June 2020

Nic was Nick's best friend all throughout elementary school and into college. They played hockey together, and after high school, Nic moved to Southern California.

Dear Savy (sorry, cannot say Nick),

There is so much to tell you since you've been gone, but there are a few things I would like to ask. The first thing is if you remember the promise we made when we were kicking back watching some Michigan football (because we had a dream to both play D1 hockey, you at Michigan and I at ND) – would you still be my best man and I yours? It seems silly, but I held that very dear to my heart because we had so many future plans to be best friends throughout our lives, and honestly bro, I miss you.

It sucks checking my phone and not getting a text, and not being able to hear your voice. It sucks not having you around. I hope you can see how I have been; how I was to finally let go of the self-hate I had the night you passed. I wish you could see my new home here in California, I wish you could meet my girlfriend who I believe I will marry, I wish you and I could have had that beer we told each other we would have on our 21st birthday (I still drink PBR on your birthday since it was the last beer we had together). At the end of the day, after all the stuff that happened in my life, good or bad, you were a constant and never left my side. You were there, you let me figure stuff out, but were not afraid to step in and help me out even when you were not asked to do so.

I miss going to the lake house and having your dad (you always called him Mike) try to blast us off the tubes, or having you trying to help me figure out how to snowboard or wakeboard, since we both knew I was so uncoordinated having my feet tied together. I miss having you as a line mate and all the parties we went to. At the end of the day, I was able to finally see who I truly was, and I was able to fight my fears and move away and truly start my own life and my own story, because I knew you were here with me. But it sucks not having my best friend by my side. I miss hearing you call everyone "Bro" or "Brah" as a term of respect. I miss hearing your "classic rock" (which was like AC/DC or Led Zeppelin) in the car so you could pass out (sleep), because let's be real – you could sleep anywhere if you had your iPod blasting those songs. I miss having you around to see the man I have become; it sucks having to do so much growing up and not have you by my side.

Some songs that always make me think of you and Jack, like when we went to the Ice Box "block party" and played "Stairway to Heaven" and any and all AC/DC songs. That was before we got into rap. Some of your sayings I miss most and have made my own:

"Life is chill, dude" and "Bro I got this." It was basic stuff but I always knew that I did not have to worry about whatever we were about to do. Having you come to all my dances in middle school, or even having my first college introduction with you by my side, are things that I will never forget. I remember before our pre-calc class my senior year, your junior year, we had to stop off at Starbucks and get some coffee, pretty much to make our teacher mad since we had the same name and could mess with him.

One thing I wish I could tell you, Savy, and to Jack, are the final words I was able to speak to you both. I love you bros. I know you are not here to see, but I actually have those tattooed on me, because you were such a huge part of my life. I will never forget the things we have been through. I love you both so much and I only wish I was able to share how much I have grown and to show y'all the place I call home and to have you meet my wife-to-be. I know you guys are in a better place, but I wish I could tell you how much you mean to me and my family. Love you bro.

Oh and one more thing Savy, even though you had other friends and I was and still am a hard person to get along with bc of my quirks (and I know I am not everyone's cup of tea), you never made me feel out of place. Again, I cannot thank you enough bc you always let me be me, and I became who I am and grew into the man I am now bc of you. I would not be who I am without you. Once again, love you bro. There will be two seats saved for both of you, and I cannot wait to have my first son to be named after both of you, Jackson Nicholas.

Nic

June 2020

Bryce was one of Jack's best friends growing up. Jack and Bryce played hockey together from a very young age, and they both excelled on the ice. Even off-ice, the families were close family friends.

Dear Jack (what up bro),

Not a day goes by where there is not something that happens that makes me think of you. You would not believe how much has happened over the last five years. So to catch you up, I'll start right where we left off.

I finally made it to Miami University and fulfilled my lifelong dream of playing college hockey. I decided to wear jersey number 5 in honor of you, because of how much you meant to me. I wanted to make you proud. I finally turned 21 and had my first legal beer. I always imagined having that with you, but I know you were there watching over having a "Busch Latte" (Busch Light) from up above.

Our family just moved down to Texas a couple years ago. Only a matter of time before we can convince Justin to ride a bull. I became the head coach of the club hockey team at Miami and actually coached against Justin. I know he's your little brother and you are looking out for him, but I really could've used a win instead of a tie. I guess I'll take what I can get from you.

I just graduated from Miami this year. I wish we could've made some memories during our college years because I am sure there would've been great stories to come from it. There is this song that came out by a country artist named Cole Swindell called "You Should Be Here," and every time it plays I think of you. It talks about a person who is not with you anymore, but the moment you are in reminds you of that person and makes you think how much they would've loved it. I have missed you so much over these last five years I cannot even begin to describe it. I have had my good days and my bad days, but one thing that stays consistent is the love I have for you. I'll see you again soon enough.

I love you, brother.

Bryce

June 2020

Grant was Jack's cousin, best friend, and confidant since fifth grade. He was a good, loyal friend who was always by Jack's side, and vice versa. The rest of Jack's friends quickly accepted Grant into their group, and they are all close friends to this day.

Dear Jack,

I don't even know where to start, but you have missed a lot of things that have happened since you passed away. You would be surprised at how well I have handled college at IU and how I have accepted a medical sales job. If you were here today, our friendship would be stronger than ever. Over the years, I still to this day have not had a friendship as close and as personal as the one I had with you.

I am sure you would have killed it at Ball State, and probably would be selling RV's like Big Mike. With your personality, you would have been a killer salesman. I assume you would have found your dream girl and would be living the life every 23-year-old would have wanted. I wanted to let you know that I have gotten a lot closer with Justin and he is about to complete his senior year at IU.

To this day, it still bothers me about the memories we could have made as best friends growing older. I mean, we never had the opportunity to go out to a restaurant and order a beer. You will always be my best friend. I hope you are doing well in heaven, brother.

Fly High,
Grant

♩

June 2020

Matt was a friend of both Jack and Nick from high school and was set to room with Jack at Ball State University for their freshman year in the fall of 2015.

Dear Jack,

Miss you, buddy – the world has not been the same without you and Nick here. I often think how different my time at Ball State would have been with you as my roommate and best friend throughout all of college. I always had a feeling you were looking over me at Ball State, though, which gave me some peace of mind.

I miss going up to Donnell Lake and being thrown off the tube from your driving, the long slip and slide down the hill, and all the other shenanigans. Going up to Donnell meant we would always stop at Porky's and get a slice of pizza or some chicken... never knew gas station food could be so great, haha! I can only hope that you and Nick are still playing pond hockey and whipping the boat around up there in heaven.

I'll never forget the times we would just get in the Cherokee and drive around after school or whenever we were bored.

Every time I hear "Riptide" by Vance Joy or something by Fetty Wap, I immediately think of some of the best times with you. Something so simple, yet it was always something to look forward to.

Keep looking over us brother! We love and miss you more than anything. I cannot wait to hear that laugh again! Love you.

Love, Matt

This is what I like about photographs:
they are proof that once, even if just for a
heartbeat, everything was perfect.

- JODI PICOULT

THE PHOTO BOOTH
Memories of Our Lives

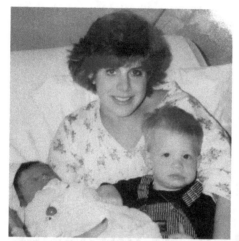

Nick meeting Jack for the first time – May 25, 1997.

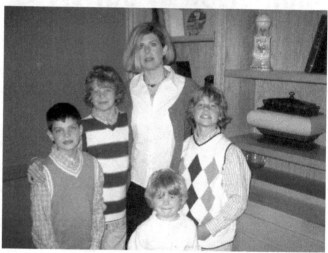

Easter brunch picture of me and my boys, 2008 (didn't we all dress our kids alike?).

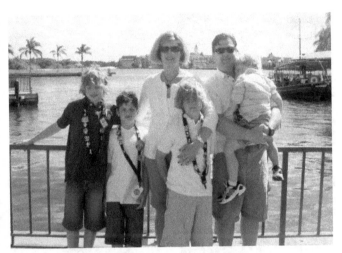

Family vacation to Disney World.

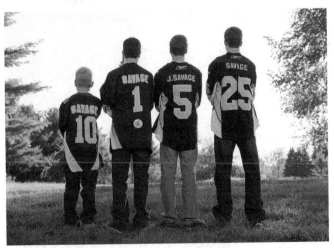

The four Savage boys in their hockey jerseys.

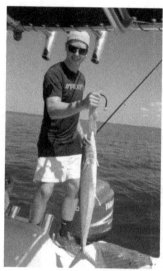

Jack, on a family
fishing trip.

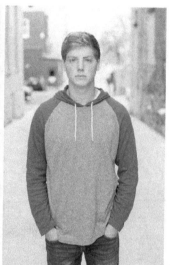

Jack's senior photo.

Not many pictures
of Nick
without Jack.

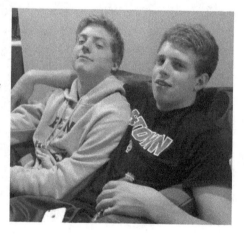

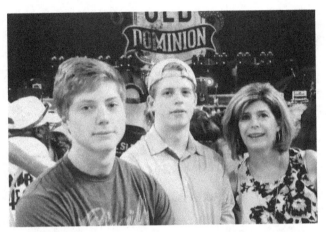

Jack, Nick and me. This picture was taken a few weeks before they passed. We were at a Kenny Chesney concert in Indianapolis, and this is where Nick heard Eric Church live and became obsessed with his album The Outsiders.

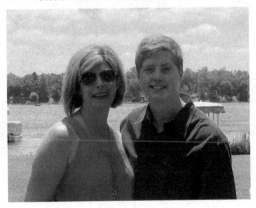

Me and Jack at his graduation party, the weekend before he passed.

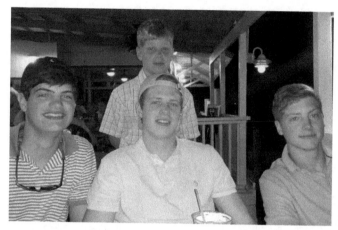

My four boys! Justin, Matthew, Nick and Jack.
This was the last picture taken of all the boys.

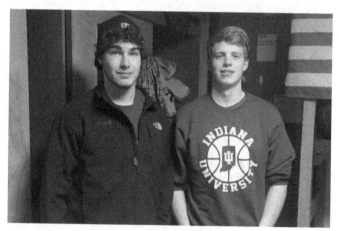

Nick's lifelong friend, Nic.

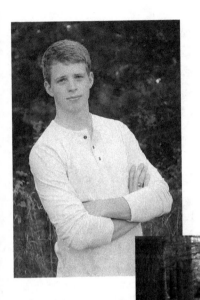

Nick's senior photo.

Nick's senior photo shoot with a few extra people! When you're a busy mom of four, you use any opportunity to grab a group photo!

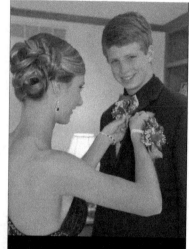

*Nick getting ready for
the senior prom.*

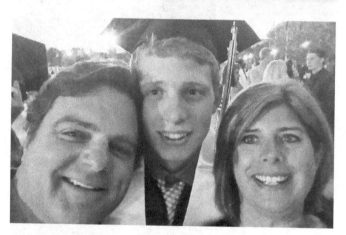

*Mike, Nick and me at Nick's high school graduation!
We were so proud of him.*

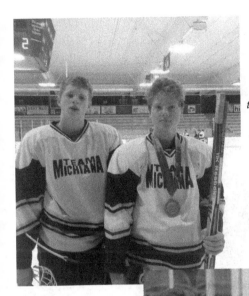

Nick and Jack shared a love for the game of hockey. Here they are playing together. (You can tell they are excited that I jumped on the ice for a quick picture after the game… not!)

Jack accepted the first-place State award for his team after they won the state championship his senior year. Jack was the team captain. Mike was the state representative for the tournament and was able to present Jack with the award!

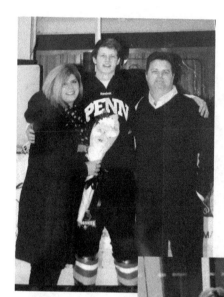

Nick on his senior night of hockey.

Jack on his senior night of hockey.

Becky

When someone we love dies, part of us
stops existing; somewhere within our
journey, we must grieve a loss of self.

When Nick graduated high school in 2014 and left
for his freshman year of college at Indiana University,
I remember being so proud of him. I remember
thinking he had so much life ahead of him. Then
Jack graduated the following year in 2015, and was
so excited to leave for Ball State that fall. I envisioned

them earning degrees, getting married, and starting big, crazy families of their own.

I had no idea that 2015 would be the year that I would say goodbye to both of them, on the same day.

But I do not want Nick and Jack to be remembered for how they died. I want them to be remembered for how they lived. And they lived their lives taking care of others, doing good deeds, and contributing to our community. They were good brothers, good sons, and good friends.

In fact, the day after they died, after spending the night at our lake house, we headed back to "the house." It was so hard to be there that day, but that is where our family and friends were gathered, and we needed them. We had only been there a short time before the doorbell rang; someone answered, and then called me to the door. There were two boys standing there, holding the biggest bouquet of flowers. I listened as they introduced themselves, and told us that they drove all night to be there...

"Mrs. Savage, these are for you," one said, as he handed me the flowers and the card.

"I went to middle school with Jack. He sat with me on the bus when no one else would sit with me. Up until that point, the kids on the bus picked on me. But when Jack sat with me and became my friend, no one ever picked on me again. That was the kind of kid Jack was, and I just wanted to tell you that story, and tell you how sorry I am for your loss."

I gave him a big hug and cried. He handed me the card and bouquet of flowers and headed back towards his home in Ohio. Hearing that story at that time was exactly what my heart needed to hear.

Stories are the way we remember our loved ones. And telling Nick and Jack's story is so important to me, because this is how their legacy lives on. We can never change what happened in the past, but we can change the future. And by telling their story, we can leave a positive legacy in Nick and Jack's name – a legacy of love, making a difference and saving lives.

Moving forward has been a progress over perfection kind of thing. I am getting better at learning to embrace and lean into the grief. Now, when I remember my older boys, I smile more often than I cry. I feel them close to me in such comforting ways. And I am reminded they are with us every day, even when they are not in my arms where I want them to be.

The 525 Foundation

The name of the foundation we started in Nick and Jack's names was inspired by a photo we had of all four boys, standing in a line, wearing their hockey jerseys. Nick and Jack were side by side in the photo. Jack was wearing the number 5 on his hockey jersey and Nick was wearing the number 25, so we called it the 525 Foundation. Since the start of the foundation in 2016, exactly one year after that fatal night in June, I have been working with lawmakers on legislation for safe drug disposal, and I have been partnering with local and national grocery stores, pharmacies and community centers to provide drug disposal drop boxes. But the most important part of this work has been sharing our message by speaking to students, parents, educators, coaches, lawmakers and first-responders about the dangers of prescription drug misuse and abuse. I have also been championing the idea that every home, every emergency vehicle, and every school should carry a few doses of Narcan (naloxone).

And about those prescription pills – as a nurse, I am not against pain medication if people need it. But I am all for being responsible with medication and disposing of it properly after it is no longer needed. I am also trained to save people's lives. Because I did not have a chance to save Nick and Jack, I am channeling that passion and that grief into saving the lives of thousands of students who are faced with the same kind of peer pressure and the same kind of choice as Nick and Jack were. The reality is, on the night of that fatal graduation party, a total of five people took pills brought to the party. They all overdosed. Three survived. Nick and Jack died.

Nick and Jack are still a part of our everyday lives. They come up in conversation all the time with our two younger sons, Justin and Matt. Sometimes the conversations are serious, and other times they are goofy – remembering the silly situations Nick and Jack were constantly in. Their friends still come around and keep in touch. This is helpful on the days when I am wracked with grief and feel like I am losing my mind. *Could we have done anything differently? Did we do the right things as parents?* But their friends – who are now beautiful, mature young adults – are the reality checks, and reminders of the good lives Nick and Jack lived. Both had hearts of gold.

Nothing will ever change the outcome of that night, So, I have had to let go of casting any blame, and I have stopped trying to beat myself up over wanting to know who brought pills to the party that night. I have had to stop trying to figure out what **actually** transpired that night, because no matter what I find out, the outcome of that night will not change. So I have chosen to focus on the things I **can** change.

Now, every single time I stand in front of a group of people to share Nick and Jack's story, I remind myself, *There is a Nick or Jack out there somewhere.* I focus on telling our story so that heartstrings and emotions are felt and tugged; so that when these teens are faced with a decision, like Nick and Jack were, they will make a better choice. Because, ultimately, it can be that **#onechoice** that makes all the difference. There are teens all across the US who are unaware of how **#onechoice** can impact their lives. They're not aware that trying something one time can be deadly, or how they are protected if they see someone in need of help. We want to empower these teens to be the difference.

The same thing can be said for the parents. Every time I stand in front of a group of people, I am also aware that there are parents, educators, coaches and caregivers – **just like I was** – out there. These are the people who ask me, "Where are the teens getting the medications from?" or they are the parents who think, *My kids would never do something like this.*

Don't turn a blind eye to this epidemic; educate yourselves on what is out there, have those conversations with your kids, and please don't ever think something like this won't happen to you – because it can. After one of my talks, I received an email from a mom who said, "Every time my kids – who are now teens and young adults – head out the door to hang out with friends, especially when I know they are going to a party, I yell, 'Remember 525!' and they know exactly what I mean."

May we all remember 525 and make better choices every day.

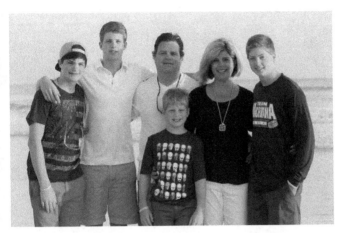

We took a family photo every year while on vacation in Siesta Key.
This was the last picture we took as a family of six.

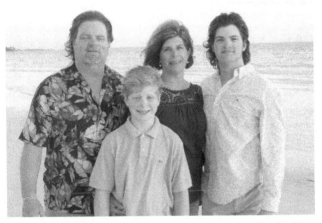

Another family photo; same beach on Siesta Key. Now a family of four.
(This is a good visual of how one bad choice can impact a whole family.)

For Teens

I am so glad that you made it this far in the book! I know it's difficult in today's world to stay away from drugs, especially when they are so commonly referred to in popular music, glamorized on social media, and are available almost anywhere you go.

Thank you for taking the time to read this book and educate yourself. In this next section, I want to give you an overview of common drugs and their effects, warnings about overuse, and a summary of overdose symptoms. I also want to share what you can do to help keep yourself and your friends safe.

I hope that you'll realize that using drugs just one time can be fatal. Please use these resources, share them with friends, and have a conversation with a trusted adult. You are worth it!

Common Drugs Used By Teens

ALCOHOL

What is it?

This is a substance that is one of the most frequently used drugs among teens. According to the National Institute on Alcohol Abuse and Alcoholism, it's one of the most abused drugs by adults, too.

How is it used?

Drinking alcohol is the most common way to use it. However there are trends which include alcohol absorption through the eyes, and using alcohol as a enema. Teens might start drinking alcohol because it makes them feel good at first or like they can escape their problems for a while. But just like any other substance, it can have negative effects on your health.

Warnings

Alcohol affects a teen's brain differently than it does an adult's. Teens' brains are still growing and developing in ways that shape their perceptions of emotions, excitement, danger, and some memories. Heavy alcohol use during this earlier time of brain development could lead to permanent changes. (Parents, this is one of those facts you are going to want to share with your teen!)

Also… there is a popular trend called alcohol blackout – this is when a teen drinks so much alcohol in a short period of time that they experience gaps in memory. Blacking out is different from passing out. A blackout is a loss of the ability to make memories; however, people are still conscious when they're blackout drunk.

ANABOLIC STEROIDS

What are they?

Anabolic steroids are drugs that are made to mimic the male hormone, testosterone. They can be prescribed legally to help with some health issues.

How are they used?

Some people who misuse these steroids take pills; others use needles to inject steroids into their muscles, or apply them to the skin as a gel or cream. Bodybuilders and athletes might misuse anabolic steroids in attempts to build muscles and improve athletic performance.

Warnings

Teens who misuse steroids have a greater risk for injury to muscles and tendons. They are also at an increased risk for heart issues, blood clots and strokes. Acne, premature balding or hair loss, weight gain, and mood swings are all side effects.

Common street names

Arnolds, juice, pumpers, roids, stackers, and weight gainers.

COCAINE

What is it?

Cocaine is a very addictive stimulant (speeds you up) that's made from the leaves of a coca plant. It comes in a white powder and is often mixed with other substances. Cocaine is so addictive that you could become addicted after your first time using it.

How is it used?

Cocaine in the powder form can be snorted up the nose or mixed with water and injected with a needle. Cocaine can also be made into small white rocks, called crack. Crack is smoked in a small glass pipe.

Warnings

Cocaine is a drug that can wear off very quickly, so it is often followed up with another use, making it easy to lose track of how much has been taken. In larger doses, it can cause anxiety, paranoia, and erratic – sometimes violent – behavior. Cocaine is also a very dangerous drug... and a ONE-TIME use CAN be FATAL! Cocaine, because it is a stimulant, speeds up your heartbeat which can lead to stroke, heart attack, and again… DEATH. Some signs of an overdose include (but are not limited to) high body temperature, profuse sweating, irregular heartbeat, chest pain, and severe confusion or delirium. If you notice ANY of these signs, please call 911 and stay with the person until help arrives. Nosebleeds, a chronic runny nose or sniffling regularly can indicate that a child has been taking the drug by snorting it. Someone buzzed on cocaine may be wide awake for long periods of time, and then fall asleep for long periods as well. This drug is popular in college towns and is related to students binge-studying.

Common street names
Street names for this drug include coke, snow, dust, powder, nose candy, coco, blow, pearl, yeyo.

Often represented with the following emojis:

DXM

What is it?

Dextromethorphan or DXM is found in most cold and flu medications at our local pharmacies or grocery stores. DXM can come in the form of syrup, cold and cough tablets, or liquid gel tabs.

How is it used?

Drinking cough syrup mixed with soda pop (a combination called "lean" or "sizzurp") has become increasingly popular among youth in several areas of the country. DXM is abused in high doses in order to experience euphoria and visual and auditory hallucinations. When ingested in large quantities, the cough suppressant can deliver a powerful buzz – a practice also known as "robotripping." Some teens use it with alcohol or marijuana or prescription medications to increase the effects.

Common street names

CCC, dex, DXM, poor man's PCP, robo, rojo, skittles, triple C, and velvet.

HEROIN

What is it?

Heroin is a street opioid narcotic (pain relieving drug). Heroin is illegal and a HIGHLY addictive drug.

How is it used?

Heroin is usually injected or smoked; sometimes, it is inhaled. Heroin provides a burst or rush of good feelings, and users feel "high" and relaxed. Those feelings may be followed by drowsiness and nausea. Most heroin users do not start with heroin; most have a prescription opioid dependency, and have switched over to heroin because it is cheaper.

Warnings

Heroin is highly addictive. People who use heroin regularly can develop a tolerance, which means that they need higher and/or more frequent doses of the drug to get the effect they crave. Heroin is also "cut" or mixed with other unknown substances. There is a high risk for overdose with heroin. When people overdose on heroin, their breathing often slows or stops. Other signs of overdose include (but are not limited to) bluish-colored lips or nails, a weak pulse, pinpoint pupils, extreme drowsiness, and repeated loss of consciousness. If any of these symptoms are noted, call 911, turn the person on their side, and wait for medical help to arrive. DO NOT leave the person alone to "sleep it off."

Common street names
Big H, black tar, hell dust, horse, smack, tar, junk, black, dragon, white horse, skag, and thunder.

Often represented by the following emojis:

INHALANTS

What are they?
Inhalants are anything that contains a fume that can create a high. They are usually found in household products and are inexpensive, making them easy for teens to obtain. Common items include glue, lighter fluid, cleaning fluids, hair spray, nail polish remover, and paint. All of these produce chemical vapors that can be inhaled.

How are they used?

People who abuse inhalants breathe in the fumes through their nose or mouth, usually by "sniffing," "snorting," "bagging," or "huffing." It is called different names depending on the substance and equipment used. Inhalants cause a sense of euphoria for about 15-45 minutes (depending on what was huffed). Teens use Inhalants because they are cheap and readily available. They can walk into any store and purchase without questions. They are fast-acting, and the effects are short-lived so they are not easily detected by parents.

Warnings

Inhalants can cause death, even after just one use! Inhalants can cause a user's heart to beat more irregularly and then stop; other effects include asphyxiation, suffocation, choking, seizures and falling into a coma. Parents, these effects are real and can happen to your child… Have that talk!

Common street names

Gluey, huff, rush, and whippets.

MARIJUANA

What is it?

Marijuana is a dry, shredded mix of flowers, stems, seeds, and leaves from the cannabis sativa plant. The mixture is usually green, brown, or gray in color and may resemble tobacco.

How is it used?

There are a few different ways people use marijuana:

- Smoking hand-rolled cigarettes called joints or marijuana cigars called blunts.

- Inhaling smoke, using glass pipes or water pipes called bongs.

- Inhaling vapor, using devices that pull the active ingredients (including THC) from the marijuana into the vapor. This is more popular with marijuana extracts/concentrates. Usually smoked with a pipe or "rig."

- Drinking tea brewed with marijuana or eating foods with marijuana cooked into them, which are sometimes called edibles. Such foods include brownies, cookies, or candy.

Marijuana affects the pleasure portion of the brain, so teens often use it to feel "good" or to feel "better." Like alcohol, marijuana is legal in a lot of states, so there is a perception that it is safe. It's relatively easy to get, and some teens report that consequences aren't as strict for being caught with marijuana as opposed to other drugs.

Warnings

There are many research articles out there related to the effects of marijuana and the developing brain. But the bottom line is that marijuana today is about four to seven times more potent than it was 20 to 25 years ago. That means the effect it has on a developing brain is that much more harmful. Marijuana is also known as the gateway drug, which means that teens who use it are more likely to try other substances. Please do your research on this drug, stick to the facts, and have those conversations.

Common street names

Aunt Mary, BC bud, blunts, boom, chronic, dope, gangster, ganja, grass, hash, herb, hydro, indo, joint, kif, Mary Jane, mota, pot, reefer, sinsemilla, skunk, smoke, weed, and yerba.

Often represented by the following emojis:

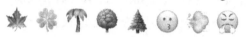

MARIJUANA EXTRACTS/CONCENTRATE

A marijuana concentrate is a highly potent concentrated form of THC (tetrahydrocannabinol) that is similar in appearance to honey or butter, and commonly referred to on the street as "honey oil" or "budder."

Marijuana concentrate can have THC levels that range from 40 to 80 percent.

Smoking or vaping it (also called dabbing) can deliver dangerous amounts of THC and has led some people to seek treatment in the emergency room.

Common street names

710 (the word "OIL" flipped and spelled backwards), wax, ear wax, butane hash oil, butane honey oil (BHO), shatter, dabs (dabbing), black glass, and errl.

METHAMPHETAMINE (METH)

What is it?

Meth is a man-made stimulant drug. It is a powder that can be made into a pill or a shiny rock (called a crystal). The rocks can be clear crystal chunks or shiny blue-white pieces.

Meth also has dangerous effects, like raising the heart rate and blood pressure, and use can lead to addiction.

How is it used?

The powder can be eaten or snorted up the nose. It can also be mixed with liquid and injected with a needle. Crystal meth is smoked in a small glass pipe. Meth produces euphoric effects — a rush of good feelings, increased energy, loss of inhibition and increased sociability. Sometimes this sense of well-being can last up to 24 hours. Methamphetamine is inexpensive and relatively easy to produce, making it affordable and readily available to teenagers.

Warnings

Meth use is associated with many serious physical problems. Since the drug is a stimulant, it can cause rapid heart rate, increased blood pressure, and damage to the small blood vessels in the brain – which could lead to a stroke! Long-term use of this drug can result in inflammation of the heart lining. Overdoses of meth can cause hyperthermia (elevated body temperature), convulsions, seizures, and death.

People who abuse meth also may have episodes of violent behavior, paranoia, anxiety, confusion, and insomnia. Meth also can cause psychotic symptoms that can last for months, or even years (even after a person has stopped using it)! Long-term use of this drug can cause teeth to decay. There is also a symptom called "bugs," where the user feels like they have bugs under their skin; so, they pick at it… not a good time!

Common street names

Rocks, crystal, crank, chalk, tweak, tina, Walter White, speed.

Often represented by the following emojis:

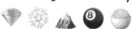

MDMA (ECSTASY OR MOLLY)

What is it?

MDMA is a man-made drug that is both a stimulant (speeds you up) and a hallucinogen (distorts a person's perception of what is real).

How is it used?

MDMA or Ecstasy is usually sold as a tablet or capsule that is swallowed. It may also be sold in powder form. The tablets may be crushed and then snorted.

The tablets come in different shapes, sizes and colors; they are often stamped with a logo, such as a butterfly or clover, giving them a candy-like look. This can be dangerous to younger teens, as they often look very similar to popular real candy.

This drug can produce feelings of pleasure and well-being, increased sociability and closeness with others. Like all stimulant drugs, MDMA/ecstasy can make users feel full of energy and confidence.

Warnings

MDMA/Ecstasy can be dangerous. Since it is a stimulant, overheating and heart issues can be a concern. As with any illegal street drug, the purity and strength can never be accurate, so when you take this, you really do not know what you are taking!

Common street names

X, Superman, XTC, Adam, beans, love drug, happy pill, Scooby snacks, Smarties, Skittles, vitamin E, or X.

Often represented by the following emojis:

   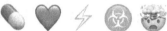

NICOTINE

What is it?

Nicotine is an addictive drug in tobacco products and e-cigarettes with both stimulant and depressant effects.

How is it used?

People can smoke, chew, or sniff tobacco products, or inhale their vapors. Smoking may make teens feel confident and provide a common ground for interacting with like-minded teens — a way to instantly bond with a group of teens. Smoking cigarettes can be a form of rebellion to flaunt their independence.

Warnings
Some of the health risks associated with tobacco use include: infertility, COPD (chronic obstructive pulmonary disease), asthma, lung cancer, heart disease, mouth and esophageal cancer, and stroke.

Common street names
E-cigs, e-hookahs, mods, vape pens, vapes, tank systems, and Juuls/Juuling.

OPIOIDS

What are they?
Opioids, sometimes called narcotics, are a large group of pain-relieving drugs that include prescription pain relievers, such as oxycodone, hydrocodone, fentanyl and tramadol. The illegal drug heroin is also an opioid.

How are they used?
When used **as directed by your doctor,** prescription opioid medications can safely help control pain, such

as pain you may have after surgery. There are risks, though, when the medications are used incorrectly.

Warnings

Anytime a prescription opioid is taken in any way other than prescribed, it can be dangerous, and can lead to death. Opioids should **never** be mixed with alcohol.

There is a high chance of overdose or death when someone misuses prescription opioids or heroin.

PRESCRIPTION MEDICATION

What are they?

Prescription medication abuse is the fastest-growing drug problem in the United States. Such abuse is the use of prescription medication in a manner that is not prescribed by a health care practitioner. That includes using someone else's prescription, or using your own prescription in a way not directed by your doctor.

How are they used?

Prescription medication abuse occurs when someone takes a medication in any other way than how it was prescribed. If someone takes two pills at a time and only one was prescribed, that's misuse. If someone takes someone else's medication, that's misuse. If someone crushes a pill and snorts it, when it was prescribed to be taken orally, that's misuse. It may be hard to imagine, but there is a lot of prescription medication misuse and abuse going on.

Prescription drugs are **only** safe for the people who have prescriptions for them.

There is a misperception that prescription drugs are safer and less harmful to one's body than other kinds of drugs, because they were prescribed by a doctor. These medications are also very easy to access without anyone noticing. Some teens take prescription drugs to get high or to experiment, often combining them with alcohol.

Warnings

Each person can react differently to taking prescription medications because our bodies break them down differently. Teens may share ADHD medications, pain pills after surgery, anxiety medications – and the list goes on and on. It is so important that we talk to our teens about the dangers of misusing prescription drugs – up to, and including, death!

Keep track of your prescription medications. Keep them in a safe and secure place and properly dispose of them when you are done with them!

SPICE/K2

What is it?
Spice or K2 refers to a class of chemicals called synthetic cannabinoids. These chemicals are made in a lab, and have effects similar to those of marijuana.

How is it used?
Most people smoke Spice by rolling it in papers (like with marijuana or handmade tobacco cigarettes); sometimes, it is mixed with marijuana. Some people also make it as an herbal tea for drinking. Others buy Spice products as liquids to use in e-cigarettes.

The effects of Spice or K2 are similar to those produced by marijuana, such as elevated mood, relaxation and altered perception. Some young people incorrectly assume that these products are "natural," and therefore harmless. There is a lot of false advertising when it comes to K2, as labeling will often indicate that the packages contain natural material.

Warnings

A common question is, "Can you die from K2?" and the answer is, "yes." The risk of overdose and death from K2 is high, because there is no way for users to know exactly which chemicals are in a dose.

Common street names

Spice, K2, blaze, paradise, demon, black magic, spike, Mr. Nice Guy, ninja, zohai, dream, genie, sence, smoke, skunk, serenity, Yucatan, fire, and crazy clown.

Other Ways Drugs Are Talked About, Using Emojis

	Can be used to mean prescription pills, drugs in general, or heroin
	A plug, i.e., a drug dealer or someone who can "hook you up" with contraband
	Smoking a joint
	Used to indicate a bong
	Can mean high-quality drugs or being very intoxicated
	"Gassed," i.e., intoxicated. Can also refer to high-quality marijuana
	To "blaze" a joint; or to be "lit," meaning intoxicated

Common Drug Slang Terms

Angel dust – PCP

Atom bomb – Marijuana mixed with heroin

Bars – Xanax

Bricks – Xanax

Bumping up – Ecstasy combined with powder cocaine

Cart – Cartridge for a vaporizer

Caviar – Taking cocaine and marijuana very closely together

Candyman – drug dealer

Dabbing – A way to inhale concentrated cannabis oil by dropping some on a hot surface and letting it vaporize

Fetty – fentanyl

Gas – Marijuana

Hulk – A 2-mg generic benzodiazepine bar

Norco – Hydrocodone

Pen – Vaping instrument for weed or tobacco; uses cartridges

Pharming – Mixing prescription drugs

Pint – Meth

Plug – Dealer

School bus – A 2-mg Xanax bar

Special K – Ketamine

Snow – Cocaine

Tweaker – someone who uses methamphetamine

Tweakin' – someone who is high on drugs and doing crazy stuff

Trapper – drug dealer

Wet – (a marijuana joint dipped in PCP)

30's – prescription drugs Percocet or Percodan (which are opioids)

What Is A Drug Overdose?

A drug overdose is taking too much of a substance – whether it is prescription, over-the-counter, legal, or illegal. Drug overdoses may be accidental or intentional. An overdose can lead to serious medical complications, including death. If you suspect that someone is overdosing, please call 911. Do not worry about getting in trouble; the most important thing is getting help for your friend. You may be the one who saves their life.

How do I know if someone is overdosing?

The exact signs of a drug overdose will vary from person to person, as different drugs and varying body chemistry can result in a variety of overdose symptoms. Common signs that someone is experiencing a drug overdose include:

Rapid heartbeat	Nausea
Increased body temperature	Vomiting
Chest pain	Confusion
Dilated pupils	Violent behavior
Difficulty in breathing	Aggression
Cessation of breath	Dizziness
Gurgling sounds (which indicate airway obstruction)	Seizures
Blue fingers or lips	Unconsciousness

A person may not experience all of these signs, but even a few of these symptoms can indicate an overdose.

Opioid Overdose Symptoms

Opioids carry a risk of overdose every time they are used. Signs of opioid overdose include:

- Slowed or shallow breathing
- A sleepy or "out of it" appearance
- Nodding off and sleeping
- Blue lips or blue fingertips and nails
- Weakened pulse
- Dry mouth and small pupils
- Confusion and lethargy
- Choking sounds or coughing when sleeping
- Unresponsiveness

If you think you may be witnessing an overdose, please call 911.

Take Action: Your Next Steps

Tips for staying safe from substance misuse and abuse:

✓ **Create an exit plan:** Have an exit plan in place if you end up in a situation that you want to get out of. For example, have a code word that you can text to your parent, so they know it is time to come and pick you up – no questions asked.

✓ **Find a friend:** Find a friend who is on the same page as you are; one that you can be a good friend to, as well.

✓ **Know the law:** In the state of Indiana, there is a law called the Lifeline Law. It can protect you from getting in trouble, if you stay on the scene and cooperate with the police by calling 911 to report a situation where someone is overdosing on drugs or alcohol. Find out if your state has a similar law.

✓ **Conversations:** Have hard conversations about prescription drugs. Conversations save lives. If you plant the seeds, they will grow. I cannot tell you how many teens have told me they changed their party plans after hearing Nick and Jack's story. There is even a mom who yells, "Remember 525!" every time her teens go to a party. Find current overdose stats at www.cdc.gov.

For Adults

If you don't have a chemistry degree and don't get a regular DEA briefing, it's nearly impossible to track all the drugs that our teens may run into out in the world. However, there are thousands of supportive resources that we can access as needed to help educate ourselves, our families, and our communities.

There are different reasons why teens use drugs and alcohol. Teens are influenced by things they see on TV, on the internet, and while using social media. Peer pressure can also be a reason for teen drug use. Sometimes teens feel like they may need to try drugs to fit in with different social groups. Drug use can also be an act of experimentation with teens, who are often curious and who also have a sense of feeling indestructible.

In addition, teens who struggle with mental health issues such as depression may use drugs to self-medicate and alleviate their symptoms.

I am a firm believer that teens should learn from their mistakes – not die. Here are some steps we can all take to make that possible.

✓ Acknowledge that there is a drug epidemic, and that everybody at some point in their lives will be impacted by it either directly or indirectly. No one is immune.

✓ Take action:
- Have important conversations with your teens.
- Clean out your medicine cabinets, dispose of unneeded medication, and move prescription pills to a safe, secure location. This is an easy step we can all take to be a part of the solution. The pills that our teens are taking most often

come from the medicine cabinet of a friend or family member. Find a drop box or pill drop campaign near you at www.dea.gov.

- Properly store your existing medications and educate yourself.

- Carry Narcan: Otherwise known as naloxone, Narcan is a nasal spray that can reverse an opioid overdose and save a life. You can get Narcan at most pharmacies without a prescription. Narcan is the safest temporary solution out on the market today.

✓ Create an exit plan with your teen and stay calm: if your teen calls you to pick them up, do not read them the riot act as soon as they get in the car. Do not ground them or keep them from their phones for months. Your disappointment is normal, but stay focused on the fact that your teen did the right thing, and that they are still alive to talk to you about it.

✓ See how you can get involved in your community.

As a parent, or other trusted adult, we can be the biggest influence in a child's life. We love them, teach them, guide them, and want to do all that we can to keep them safe. Teens need concrete reasons to avoid alcohol and other drugs. They need facts and evidence. We need to know what we are talking about if we want our teens to listen. How do we know what drugs are out there? What do they look like? What do my teens already know? Read thoroughly, educate yourself, and then have a conversation with your teens!

Please download our latest resources – Conversation Starters, the #ONECHOICE Student Study Guide, and more at www.525foundation.org, now!

A Final Thought from Becky

My sons lost everything because of **One Choice.** They were smart boys, but that **One Choice** cost them their lives, their family, their friends, and their dreams.

Learn from their mistakes.

Live the dreams you want to live.

Only **you** are able to decide who you are and who you want to be.

Becky

Acknowledgments

Thank you to the 525 Foundation staff, board members, and our partners in prevention. Special thanks to Sarah Albert for believing in our mission and working tirelessly to promote it! I am so thankful for you!

Thank you to all of the readers who will use our book as a conversation starter, with the hope of making a difference in someone's life. Knowing this makes the difficult task of putting these words to paper worth it.

Thank you, Beth Graybill, for helping me put all of my thoughts to paper and for finding Nick and Jack's voice. I am forever grateful that our paths crossed, and I realize that I could not have done this without you!

Thank you to everyone at O'Leary Publishing, especially April O'Leary and Heather Desrocher! Your constant encouragement, the hours together on Zoom, and the numerous texts and emails (sometimes daily!) to ensure that "this story needs to be told" worked! We did it, girls!! I am forever thankful for the two of you, each and every day!

To Nick, Jack, Justin and Matthew – I am forever grateful that I am blessed to be your mom. No matter what, I will always be your biggest cheerleader and will love you unconditionally. Near or far, I love you more . . . Always.

Thank you to my husband Mike, my family, my friends, and the Buttercups for realizing there isn't a time limit on grief, and for always loving me, even when I wasn't so lovable.

Finally, I want to thank God, who I have felt by my side every step of the way. On days when I felt lost, tired and defeated, He pushed me through. He knew that the time would come when I would need to share this story, and Nick and Jack would need to continue their purpose – and by doing this, countless lives would be saved.

About The Authors

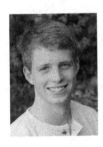

Nick Savage was a steady 19-year-old with a calm demeanor and contagious smile. He was a first-year student at Indiana University in Bloomington, Indiana, where he was majoring in chemistry and microbiology. During Nick's tenure on the hockey team at Penn High School in Mishawaka, Indiana, he led his teammates to the state runner-up title. Coaches and teammates say he led by example, both on and off the ice. Nick loved playing ice hockey, riding dirt bikes, and listening to music. Nick especially enjoyed the family lake house on Donnell Lake in southwest Michigan, where he liked to be out on the pontoon boat, or around the bonfire, with friends. Nick lost his life on June 14, 2015, due to an accidental overdose at a friend's graduation party.

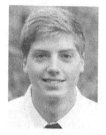

Jack Savage was an adventurous 18-year-old with a crooked smile and infectious laugh who graduated from Penn High School in Mishawaka, Indiana. Jack was captain of the state championship ice hockey team, where coaches and teammates say he led by example. Jack loved ice hockey, hunting, waterskiing, racing dirt bikes, and time around the bonfire. His favorite family pastime was wrestling with his brothers – whom he affectionately called his "bros" – and having fun with his friends at the family lake house on Donnell Lake in southwest Michigan. Jack was headed to Ball State University to major in business, until he lost his life on June 14, 2015, due to an accidental overdose at a friend's graduation party.

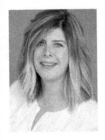 **Becky Savage** is the mother of Nick and Jack, and the co-founder of the 525 Foundation. She is a prevention specialist, and has been a registered nurse for over 30 years. She is a sought-after national speaker who educates teens, parents, first responders, and school officials on the dangers of prescription drug misuse. Becky is passionate about primary prevention through outreach, education, and support. She has a BS in nursing from Ball State University and an MS in nursing education from Bethel University. Becky and her husband Mike love spending time at Donnell Lake, Michigan with their two young adult sons, Justin and Matt. When Becky is not out on the lake or at home in Granger, Indiana, she can be found at an ice rink somewhere, or chasing her crazy dogs – Tucker, Cash, Sadie and Josie.

To book Becky to help promote prevention in your area, please visit www.beckysavage.com.